ACS SYMPOSIUM SERIES **256**

Polymeric Materials and Artificial Organs

Charles G. Gebelein, EDITOR
Youngstown State University

Based on a symposium sponsored by
the Division of Organic Coatings
and Plastics Chemistry
at the 185th Meeting
of the American Chemical Society,
Seattle, Washington,
March 20–25, 1983

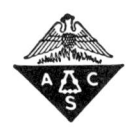

American Chemical Society, Washington, D.C. 1984

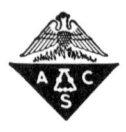

Library of Congress Cataloging in Publication Data
Polymeric materials and artificial organs.
(ACS symposium series, ISSN 0097-6156; 256)

"Based on a symposium sponsored by the Division of Organic Coatings and Plastics Chemistry at the 185th Meeting of the American Chemical Society, Seattle, Washington, March 20-25, 1983."

Bibliography: p.
Includes indexes.

1. Artificial organs—Materials—Congresses.
2. Prosthesis—Materials—Congresses. 3. Polymers in medicine—Congresses.

I. Gebelein, Charles G. II. American Chemical Society. Division of Organic Coatings and Plastics Chemistry. III. American Chemical Society. Meeting (185th: 1983: Seattle, Wash.) IV. Series.

RD130.P64 1984   617'.95   84-9297
ISBN 0-8412-0854-9

Copyright © 1984

American Chemical Society

All Rights Reserved. The appearance of the code at the bottom of the first page of each chapter in this volume indicates the copyright owner's consent that reprographic copies of the chapter may be made for personal or internal use or for the personal or internal use of specific clients. This consent is given on the condition, however, that the copier pay the stated per copy fee through the Copyright Clearance Center, Inc., 21 Congress Street, Salem, MA 01970, for copying beyond that permitted by Sections 107 or 108 of the U.S. Copyright Law. This consent does not extend to copying or transmission by any means—graphic or electronic—for any other purpose, such as for general distribution, for advertising or promotional purposes, for creating a new collective work, for resale, or for information storage and retrieval systems. The copying fee for each chapter is indicated in the code at the bottom of the first page of the chapter.

The citation of trade names and/or names of manufacturers in this publication is not to be construed as an endorsement or as approval by ACS of the commercial products or services referenced herein; nor should the mere reference herein to any drawing, specification, chemical process, or other data be regarded as a license or as a conveyance of any right or permission, to the holder, reader, or any other person or corporation, to manufacture, reproduce, use, or sell any patented invention or copyrighted work that may in any way be related thereto. Registered names, trademarks, etc., used in this publication, even without specific indication thereof, are not to be considered unprotected by law.

PRINTED IN THE UNITED STATES OF AMERICA

ACS Symposium Series

M. Joan Comstock, *Series Editor*

Advisory Board

Robert Baker
U.S. Geological Survey

Martin L. Gorbaty
Exxon Research and Engineering Co.

Herbert D. Kaesz
University of California—Los Angeles

Rudolph J. Marcus
Office of Naval Research

Marvin Margoshes
Technicon Instruments Corporation

Donald E. Moreland
USDA, Agricultural Research Service

W. H. Norton
J. T. Baker Chemical Company

Robert Ory
USDA, Southern Regional
 Research Center

Geoffrey D. Parfitt
Carnegie-Mellon University

Theodore Provder
Glidden Coatings and Resins

James C. Randall
Phillips Petroleum Company

Charles N. Satterfield
Massachusetts Institute of Technology

Dennis Schuetzle
Ford Motor Company
 Research Laboratory

Davis L. Temple, Jr.
Mead Johnson

Charles S. Tuesday
General Motors Research Laboratory

C. Grant Willson
IBM Research Department

FOREWORD

The ACS SYMPOSIUM SERIES was founded in 1974 to provide a medium for publishing symposia quickly in book form. The format of the Series parallels that of the continuing ADVANCES IN CHEMISTRY SERIES except that in order to save time the papers are not typeset but are reproduced as they are submitted by the authors in camera-ready form. Papers are reviewed under the supervision of the Editors with the assistance of the Series Advisory Board and are selected to maintain the integrity of the symposia; however, verbatim reproductions of previously published papers are not accepted. Both reviews and reports of research are acceptable since symposia may embrace both types of presentation.

CONTENTS

Preface vii

1. The Basics of Artificial Organs 1
   Charles G. Gebelein

2. Synthetic Polymeric Biomaterials 13
   Allan S. Hoffman

3. Artificial Organs and the Immune Reponse 31
   P. Y. Wang and C. Chambers

4. The Basics of Biomedical Polymers: Interfacial Factors 39
   Robert E. Baier

5. Fibrinogen-Glass Interactions: A Synopsis of Recent Research 45
   J. L. Brash, S. Uniyal, B. M. C. Chan, and A. Yu

6. Silicones in Artificial Organs 63
   E. E. Frisch

7. Characteristics of an Implantable Elastomer: Finger Joint Prosthesis
   Application 99
   H. B. Lee, H. Quach, D. B. Berry, and W. J. Stith

8. The Current Status of Prosthetic Heart Valves 111
   Ajit P. Yoganathan, E. C. Harrison, and R. H. Franch

9. Polymeric Membranes for Artificial Lungs 151
   Don N. Gray

10. Blood Compatibility of Artificial Organs: Transient Leukopenia
    in Hemodialysis 163
    S. Murabayashi and Y. Nose

11. Artificial Cells 171
    Thomas Ming Swi Chang

12. Infected Skin Wounds in Rodents: Treatment with a Hydrogel Paste
    Containing Silver Nitrate 181
    P. Y. Wang

13. Skin Regeneration with a Bioreplaceable Polymeric Template 191
    I. V. Yannas, J. F. Burke, D. P. Orgill, and E. M. Skrabut

Author Index 199

Subject Index 199

PREFACE

A HEALTHY BODY WITH PROPERLY FUNCTIONING ORGANS is a blessing that passes unnoticed by most recipients. Most people are basically unaware of the amazing chemical and physical activities that occur regularly in their bodies without any need of external stimulus or regulation. Reasonably healthy individuals rarely note the steady pulsations of the heart or the rhythmical operation of their breathing apparatus. Even the occasional demands of the body for additional fuel (food) or the expulsion of waste material (excretion) are seldom related to the operation of the organs. This basic unawareness is, of course, as it should be; the body has been designed to operate without special, overt attention. Unfortunately, this state is not true for everyone. Either through inherited defects, old age, disease, accident, or some other cause, some of the normal functionings of these organs no longer occur in the proper manner. At the least, this problem causes discomfort; at the extreme, it results in death. Approaches to dealing with this problem include medication, transplantation, life-style modification, and artificial organs. This book is concerned only with the last approach.

Artificial organs pose an enormous challenge to the scientist and to the recipient. For the recipient, the challenge is to exist and to function with a new, unnatural device that operates less effectively than a healthy organ. This difficulty is, of course, tempered by the realization that the alternatives are almost always less satisfactory. Although not normally as personal, the challenge for the scientist is also great. How can an artificial organ be designed? What materials can be used? How long will the organ function and how well will it work? What interaction will the artificial device have with the recipient? These questions are but a few that could be asked and must be answered. Some of these answers will be found in this book; some will be found elsewhere in the scientific literature; and some remain to be discovered.

Artificial organs are constructed, to a great extent, from natural or synthetic polymeric materials. In this book, we consider some of the kinds of polymeric materials used in some artificial organs. Not every material tried is described nor are all potential organs discussed in any detail. We have attempted to overview the field and to illustrate the approaches that are used and the problems that remain unsolved. Entire books have been written about a single artificial organ or polymeric material, and hundreds of papers on these subjects are published in scientific journals each year. Unfortunately, these articles appear in an extremely broad range of journals; some of these journals are highly specialized and are, therefore, almost unknown to researchers outside the immediate discipline. To be successful, however, an artificial organ must be developed by using the talents, knowledge, and input of a diverse group of scientists. This group includes chemists, chemical engineers, biologists, physicists, medical doctors, biomedical engineers, electrical engineers, and mechanical engineers, each of whom has a specialized language developed for their discipline. Developing workable artificial organs requires communication between each of these disciplines. The 13 chapters in this book, and the more than 400 references contained therein, will greatly aid neophyte and expert in this quest.

I thank each author for preparing the splendid manuscripts contributed to this volume and also the various, anonymous reviewers who helped to make these articles even better. I also thank the Division of Organic Coatings and Plastics Chemistry (now called the Division of Polymeric Materials: Science and Engineering) for their assistance and encouragement in this project. Last, but not least, I thank my family and friends for their support and encouragement in preparing this book. We all sincerely hope that it will prove useful in developing the better artificial organs of the future.

CHARLES G. GEBELEIN
Youngstown State University

April 4, 1984

The Basics of Artificial Organs

CHARLES G. GEBELEIN

Department of Chemistry, Youngstown State University, Youngstown, OH 44555

The primary purpose of this paper is to review the types of devices that are currently used in the human body as artificial organs and prosthetic devices. By definition, an organ is a specialized structure (e.g. heart, kidney, limb, leaf, flower) in an animal or a plant that can perform some specialized function. Most parts of the human body can be classed as organs. These varied parts sometimes become defective and must be replaced by an artifical organ or a prosthetic device. In almost all cases, these replacement devices are constructed of natural or synthetic polymeric materials. Such biomaterials must exhibit good compatibility with the blood and the body fluids and tissues with which they come into contact. In addition, the artificial device must closely duplicate the function of the natural organ. In practice, these artificial devices are constructed from a wide variety of materials such as metals, ceramics (including glass and carbon), natural tissues (actually polymeric in nature), and synthetic polymers. Partly due to the wider range of properties available, most of these artificial devices are constructed wholly or partly from natural or synthetic polymers. Obviously the same polymer could not be used for all possible artificial organs or prosthetic devices. Rather, the material to be used must be matched to the specific use requirements. Artificial organs can conveniently be classed into four groups: (I) Bone/Joint Replacements (e.g. hip, knee, finger, total limb), (II) Skin/Soft Tissue Replacements (e.g. skin, breast, muscle), (III) Internal Organs (e.g. heart, kidney, blood vessels, liver, pancreas), and (IV) Sensory Organs (e.g. eye, ear). This paper will consider the basic requirements for some of these artificial organs and will discuss the

0097-6156/84/0256-0001$06.00/0
© 1984 American Chemical Society

various polymeric materials that are used. The greatest emphasis will be on the chemistry and biomaterial requirements of the artificial internal organs.

The primary purpose of this chapter is to review the types of devices that are being used in the human body at the present time as artificial organs, prosthetic devices or general implants. Subsequent chapters in this book will consider some of these devices, etc. in more detail. In a similar manner, other papers consider the various polymeric and non-polymeric materials that are used and discuss the specialized requirements for these applications. These areas are covered in this paper only slightly since they are discussed in detail elsewhere.

An artificial organ clearly is a replacement for a natural organ in the body. The dictionary defines an organ as "a differentiated structure (as a heart, kidney, leaf, flower) in an animal or plant made up of various cells and tissues and adapted for the performance of some specific function..." Although this definition might be modified somewhat in a medical textbook, it will serve to cover and illustrate the range in applications and properties that occur in this rather specialized field. Most parts of the human body can be classed as an organ by this definition and could, potentially, be replaced by an artificial organ or by a prosthetic/biomedical device. This constitutes a very broad range of functions and properties which are often of an opposing nature and hundreds of specific devices have been tried as replacement parts, often with limited success. Part of this problem is due to the fact that the requirements for each device are highly specific and the materials used must meet these varied specifications. Obviously, the material used to replace a bone or a joint would not be a likely candidate for an artificial skin or a soft tissue replacement merely on the basis of the different physical characteristics of each type of biomaterial. Superimposed on this general requirement is the fact that the body has been designed to detect, attack and/or reject any foreign materials that come into contact with the bodies tissues and most synthetic materials are not compatible with the various tissues, fluid and the blood of the human body. Natural materials, on the other hand, usually elicit an even more severe rejection response from the body although some natural tissues have been modified by various chemical treatments which enable them to be tolerated to some extent (e.g. treatment of replacement porcine heart valves with glycerol or an aldehyde). This problem is especially evident in the related area of organ transplantation. Partly for this reason, essentially all the artificial organs, prosthetic devices and/or implants are made from ceramics (which could also include various glasses and some special forms of carbon), metals or synthetic polymers. Because the polymeric materials (both natural and synthetic) have a wider range of properties that are needed in these varied applications, and because they are also more compatible, in some cases, with the body tissues than the other classes of materials, polymers are the most widely used type of material in this field.

It is not possible to cover all aspects of artificial organs in this short paper and further information and references can be found in some recent review articles and books (1-18). In this paper we will outline the nature of the devices and materials currently used as artificial organs. For convenience these will be subdivided into the categories of: (I) Bone/Joint Replacement; (II) Skin/Soft Tissue Replacements; (III) Internal Organs; and (IV) Sensory Organs.

Type (I) - Bone/Joint Replacements

In many cases it is necessary to replace a defective joint with a prosthetic device to alleviate a condition caused by an accident or a degenerative disease. Joint replacements must meet some specific requirements including: (a) maintainance of normal joint space; (b) good, steady, natural motion; (c) firm and 'permanent' fixation; (d) readily lubricated; (e) stress and erosion resistant; and (f) biocompatibility.

Most joint replacements utilize polymers to some extent. Finger joints usually are replaced with a poly(dimethylsiloxane) insert and over 400,000 such replacements are made each year (1). More recently a poly(1,4-hexadiene) polymer has been tried in this application (1). Many other parts of the hand, such as the bones, have also been replaced by silicone rubber. Other types of joints, such as the hip or the knee, often involve the contact of a metal ball or rider on a plastic surface which is usually made from high density, high molecular weight polyethylene. These metal and plastic parts are usually anchored in the body using a 'cement' of poly(methyl methacrylate) which is polymerized *in situ*. Full and partial hip prostheses are implanted about 250,000 times annually while the knee replacement occurs about 100,000 times each year (5). The major problems that occur in joint replacement are: (a) wear with patient irritation due to the debris, and (b) loosening of the prosthesis which results in unsteady motion and increased wear (1, 19, 20). In some cases, injury, genetic defects or sickness requires the complete or partial replacement of an upper or lower limb. The difficulty of obtaining an adequately working prosthesis increases markedly with the amount of the limb that must be replaced. In other words, it is more difficult to design a satisfactory prosthesis for an arm than for a hand. In addition, functional lower limb replacements are more difficult to achieve than are upper limb replacements. This is due, in part, to the fact that while many of the upper limb functions can be done with only one limb, the primary function of the lower limbs, walking, cannot. A number of partial or total prostheses do, however, exist for lower limb replacement which can be utilized to permit a reasonable degree of locomotion. Some of these devices utilize hydraulic knee joints as part of the design (21-24). Upper limb replacement can be either cosmetic and/or functional. Normally when only one upper limb is replaced, the patient does the majority of limb functions with the other limb, even when this had been the non-dominant arm, because the artificial limb does not function nearly as well as the natural one. The more recent myoelectric activated devices show much promise toward duplicating the function of a natural arm or hand but much remains to be done in this area (24-26).

Type (II) - Skin/Soft Tissue Replacement

The skin is the largest organ in the body from the standpoint of weight or volume. At the present time there is no material that can duplicate this complex organ in all its functions but over 100,000 people are hospitalized annually with severe skin damage (burns, accidents, etc.) that requires immediate treatment to prevent gross bacterial contamination and/or the loss of body fluids and electrolytes. The most promising approach to this problem has utilized a composite system consisting of a collagen-glycosaminoglycan inner membrane with a silicone rubber outer layer (27). Other approaches have included dextran hydrogels (28), various polypeptides (29), and collagen (30). These materials attempt to duplicate the barrier properties of the skin with good success, but no material has yet been able to duplicate the other skin functions and a true artificial skin does not yet exist.

A large portion of the human body is composed of soft tissues including muscles, fatty tissues and connective tissues. The general area of plastic and/or reconstructive surgery involves this type of tissue to a large extent. Each year there are at least 200,000 breast prostheses and/or augumentations (7), 200,000 facial plastic surgeries (1), and 35,000 hernia repairs conducted (15). A satisfactory soft tissue material must have suitable long-term, physical properties (soft and/or rubbery), and not cause any adverse effect in the patient. Very few materials can meet these general (and some other specific) requirements. For example, sponges and textiles might have suitable "softness" but the ingrowth of fibrous tissue quickly renders these materials unsatisfactory since the implant becomes more rigid or hard after this ingrowth. While many materials have been tried for soft tissue replacement, the most common one is poly(dimethylsiloxane) which can be made in the form of rubbery gels, tubes and/or sheets with varying degrees of 'stiffness' produced by varying levels of crosslinking. Some limited use has been found for polyethylene, polyurethane and the synthetic rubbers (1, 15, 31-33).

Type (III) - Internal Organs

The area of artificial internal organs includes the heart, lungs, liver, kidneys, pancreas, blood vessels and the gastro-intestinal tract. In addition to the obvious requirements of blood and tissue compatibility, these replacements often have highly specialized functions which are almost impossible to duplicate with man-made materials. Nevertheless, it is often necessary to augment or replace the function of these organs.

Over 100,000 pacemakers are implanted annually to regulate the heart beat and these devices are usually polymer coated to protect the electronic portions from the body fluids. Pacemakers have been used experimentally in animals since 1932 and have been used in humans since 1952 to treat Stokes-Adams disease (heart block). Implantable pacemakers were first used in 1958. The more recent versions of these devices are capable of varying the heart beat rate (34, 35).

While there are four valves in the heart, almost all the replacements are done on either the aortic or mitral valves. A wide variety of designs have been devised for these valve replacements utilizing many natural and synthetic polymers. The major types of materials used are porcine valves, which have been pretreated with glycerol or an aldehyde to reduce immune responses, polymeric materials, such as silicone rubber, tetrafluoroethylene and Dacron®, metals and some ceramics (especially certain types of carbon). The most common designs for the devices using synthetic polymers contain a ball in a cage or some form of a disc in a cage. In some cases, human dura mater has been utilized as a valve material. Over 30,000 heart valve replacements are made annually. In nearly all cases, the patient must receive regular anti-coagulant medication for the remainder of their life in order to avoid blood clots (1, 30, 36-38).

In 1980, over 110,000 coronary artery bypass operations were performed in the United States alone (5). In addition, there were a large number of other blood vessel replacements and/or repairs done with the total being in excess of 200,000. While much of this surgery is done using natural materials (autogeneous blood vessels when possible), a large portion of this surgery utilizes synthetic polymers. These are usually Dacron®, in the form of knitted or woven tubes, or polytetrafluoroethylene, in the form of a 'micro-expanded tube.' While the natural blood vessels might seem preferable, in cases of advanced disease the other vessels of the body are often defective and would not be suitable replacement materials. A good example would be the saphenous veins, which are commonly used in heart bypass surgery, but frequently are too weak or blocked to be used in some patients. For this reason synthetic materials are essential. The use of woven or knitted Dacron® blood vessel prostheses dates from the pioneering work of DeBakey in 1951 and this material is frequently the prosthesis of choice among many heart surgeons

(39). These Dacron® prostheses can only be used for vessels 6 mm or larger. The mode of operation involves implanting the prosthesis whose open pores rapidly become filled or clogged with a thrombus (blood clot) which is then gradually replaced by a new tissue called neointima. It is this neointima that eventually contacts the blood rather than the thrombogenic Dacron®. The neointima appears to be similar in its composition to the natural blood vessel material. In tubes much smaller than 6 mm, the neointima blocks off the vessel to a great extent.

The use of expanded tetrafluoroethylene (PTFE) prostheses (Gore-Tex®) has permitted the replacement of vessels as small as 4 mm. The neointima layer is thinner in this system. Experimental work in dogs has used PTFE vessels as small as 3 mm successfully (40, 41). Unfortunately, most of the blood vessels in the human body are smaller than this size and no suitable material is yet available although many experimental materials show considerable promise. These include various hydrogels (12) and certain polyether polyurethane ureas (PEUUs) (42, 43).

Over a million deaths occur annually in the USA due to heart disease and over 500,000 are hospitalized each year with heart attacks (1). Certainly one of the most spectacular type of operations involves the total replacement of the heart. Most generally, this is done by means of a transplant from a human donor. For obvious reasons, the replacement organ is not readily available. Animal hearts (or other organs) are rapidly rejected by the human body. Much research has been done to develop a total artificial heart (TAH) or a partial assist device (left ventricular assist device; LVAD) and some success has been achieved in this area. For example, cows have been kept alive for over seven months with a TAH. In most cases, the TAH consists of a pair of LVADs. The LVAD itself is designed to permit a partial rest for a working heart and thereby permit healing to occur more readily. While the LVADs and TAHs are usually implanted, the devices are powered and controlled externally. Many different polymeric materials have been tried in these devices, but the most widely used one, at present, is a polyether polyurethane which is used in the pumping diaphram and the lining of the pump chamber which contacts the blood. This polyether polyurethane has fair blood compatibility and does show sufficient durability to undergo the 36+ million flexings which would occur in a blood pump each year of use. (Most materials cannot achieve this value; the desired duration of use is projected to be at least ten years, or 360+ million flexings.) Other synthetic polymers that have been tried for this application include silicone rubber, polyvinylchloride (plasticized), natural rubber and some synthetic rubbers such as poly(1,4-hexadiene).

The TAH has been used three times in humans. In the first two cases (1969 and 1981) the TAH was used to maintain life until a heart transplant could be made a few days later. The third case, Dr. Barney Clark, involved the permanent replacement of the human heart with the TAH, and the device kept him alive for about three additional months. (Death was due to other causes rather than failure of the TAH.) It is highly likely that this, or similar devices, will be used many times in the future (1, 11, 45-47).

The most widely used heart assist device, other than the heart-lung machine routinely used in surgery, is the intraaortic balloon pump (IABP) which consists of a PEUU balloon mounted on a hollow catheter. The IABP is inserted into the aorta via the femoral artery and is then expanded and contracted by an external pumping system to match the heart beat. While this device does provide significant improvement in circulation and also allows the heart to rest partially after a myocardial infarction, the mortality rate is still 65-90% (48).

Over 40,000 people in the United States, and over 100,000 people worldwide, were maintained on dialysis units in 1982 (1). In addition, many others were placed on this device, which is commonly called an artificial kidney, for brief periods of time in order to correct a temporary problem. The artificial kidney is an extracorporeal device which consists of a dialysis membrane unit and various tubing, pumping and regulating equipment, which is used to remove the waste materials from the blood and thereby mimics the operation of a healthy kidney. The preferred treatment for a defective kidney is actually transplantation, which was first done in 1954. Although a person can function satisfactorily with only one kidney, a transplanted organ will be rejected by the recipient unless careful tissue matching is done. While the newer immunosuppressant drugs, such as cyclosporin, have aided greatly in permitting greater success in organ transplantation, the number of available organs remains well below the demand. For this reason alone, many patients remain on dialysis for many years. In recent years, portable or wearable devices have been developed which allow the patient considerable mobility compared with the past but the dialysis device leaves much to be desired as an ideal replacement for the kidney. Unfortunately, it appears unlikely that a satisfactory, implantable 'true' artificial kidney will be developed in the near future. The present devices utilize polymers in the tubing (usually silicone rubber, poly (vinyl chloride) or polyethylene; the tubing is either treated with heparin or heparin is added to the blood during use to prevent clotting) and in the membrane itself (usually cellulosic although polyacrylonitrile has been used in the hollow fiber type) (1, 9, 11, 17).

The pancreas serves several functions which includes the secretion of the enzyme insulin which controls blood glucose metabolism level. Over a million diabetic persons must take insulin injections on a regular basis (1). The metabolism control by this method is erratic and several research groups have been experimenting with polymeric infusion pumps in order to control the insulin level (and thus the glucose level) more closely. If such a device would be coupled with an implanted glucose sensor, the extent of control could approach that of a healthy pancreas, except for insulin synthesis (1, 49).

No implantable, artificial lungs exist at this time but some research has been done on polymeric membranes that could be used in such a device. Extracorporeal blood oxygenators are, however, used in excess of 100,000 times a year (1) and contain a thin, polymeric membrane thru which O_2 and CO_2 are exchanged. These oxygenators, which exist in several different styles are widely used in by-pass and other operations. The main polymers used are silicone rubber but poly(alkylsulfones) and some others show promise (1, 50, 51).

The liver is the main detoxification organ in the body and therefore comes into contact with nearly every poison and toxin that enters the body. These materials could occur in case of poisoning, drug overdose, acute hepatitis, and allergies. While no true artificial liver has been developed, and transplantation is rare and difficult, several approaches have been attempted to replace and/or assist the function of the liver. The most common method is hemoperfusion in which the blood is passed through a column or bed of some sorbent material which can remove the poisons. The sorbents that have been used include charcoal, ion-exchange resins, affinity chromatography resins, immobilized enzymes and hepatic material or pieces of liver enclosed in 'artificial cells' (9, 52).

Various types of plastic tubing have been used to replace sections of the gastro-intestinal tract or other tube-like parts of the body. These seldom have any function other than connecting one part of the body with the other. Because of the complex variety of chemical operations involved, it is unlikely that a true artificial GI tract will be developed in the near future (1,15).

Type (IV) - Sensory Organs

Polymeric materials have been used to replace the external part of the ear (usually silicones) and also to replace the ossicles (PTFE, polyethylene, silicones) as well as serving as drainage tubes for the ear (11). In addition some research has been done in which electrodes are implanted into the cochlea and are connected to an external microphone. Such devices have been able to restore a significant amount of hearing to deaf people. Plastics are used in these primarily as coatings for the wires and electronic parts (14, 53, 54).

The most common use of polymeric materials in the eye is in contact lenses which are worn by several million people. Most soft contact lenses are hydrogels made from homo- or copolymers of hydroxyethyl methacrylate; hard contacts are usually made from poly (methyl methacrylate). Intraocular lenses are put into about 600,000 people annually (5). These are usually made from poly (methyl methacrylate) although hydrogels are being explored for this use (55). Some research is also being done to enable a blind person to have some 'sight' by direct stimulation of the visual area of the brain with electrodes connected to a TV type camera. At the present, this is limited to the creation of small points of light (14, 53, 56).

Little, if any, research is being conducted on the senses of smell, touch or taste that involves polymers.

In conclusion, we note that many types of artificial organs have been developed using a variety of polymeric materials but all these devices are generally less satisfactory than the original, healthy organ. In most cases, however, the artificial organ functions significantly better than the defective organ it replaces. Much more research is needed in this area. The ultimate solution will involve the creation of newer polymers and also better artificial organ designs.

Literature Cited

1. Gebelein, C.G., "Prosthetic and Biomedical Devices," in Kirk-Othmer Encyclopedia of Chemical Technology, 3rd ed., 1982; 19, 275-313.
2. Gebelein, C.G.; Koblitz, F.F., eds., "Biomedical and Dental Applications of Polymers," Plenum Publ. Corp., New York, 1981.
3. Carraher, C.E.; Gebelein, C.G., eds., "Biological Activities of Polymers," American Chemical Society Symposium Series No. 186, Washington, D.C., 1982.
4. Black, J., "Biological Performance of Materials. Fundamentals of Biocompatibility," Marcel Dekker, New York, 1981.
5. Hench, L.L., J. Biomed. Mater. Res., 1980; 14, 803.
6. Gebelein, C.G., Org. Coatings Plast. Chem., 1980, 42, 70.
7. Habel, M.B., Biomater. Med. Devices, Artificial Organs, 1979; 7(2), 229.
8. Park, J.B., "Biomaterials, An Introduction," Plenum Publ. Corp., New York, 1979.
9. Chang, T.M.S., "Artificial Kidney, Artificial Liver and Artificial Cells," Plenum Publ. Corp., New York, 1978.
10. White, R.L.; Meindl, J.D., Science, March, 1977; 195, 1119.
11. Kolff, W.J., Artificial Organs, 1977; 1 (1), 8.
12. Andrade, J., ed., "Hydrogels for Medical and Related Applications," American Chemical Society Symposium No. 31, Washington, D.C., 1976.
13. Gregor, H.P., ed., "Biomedical Applications of Polymers," Plenum Publ. Corp., New York, 1975.
14. Kronenthal, R.L.; Oser, Z.; Martin, E., "Polymers in Medicine and Surgery," Plenum Publ. Corp., New York, 1975.
15. Lee, H.; Neville, K., "Handbook of Biomedical Plastics," Pasadena Technology Press, Pasadena, CA, 1971.

16. Bement, Jr., A.L., ed., "Biomaterials," U. Washington Press, Seattle, 1971.
17. Gutcho, M., "Artificial Kidney Systems," Noyes Data Corp., Park Ridge, NJ, 1970.
18. Seltzer, R.J., C&EN, Nov. 15, 1982, pp. 61-63.
19. Charnley, J., Plastics & Rubber, 1976; 1, (2), 59.
20. Sonstefard, D.A.; Matthews, L.S.; Kaufer, H., Sci. Am., 1978; 238 (1), 44.
21. Tohen Z., A., "Manual of Mechanical Orthopaedics," Milam, R.W.; Lopez, E., translators, Charles C. Thomas, Springfield, IL, 1973.
22. Reswick, J.B.; Vodovnik, L. in "Future Goals of Engineering in Biology and Medicine," Dickson, III, J.F.; Brown, J.H.V., eds., Academic Press, New York, 1969, pp. 147-166.
23. Ducheyne, P. and Hastings, G.W., eds., "Fuctional Behavior Of Orthopedic Biomaterials", Vol. I and II, CRC Press, Boca Raton, FL, 1983.
24. Murphy, E.F., J. Biomed. Mater. Res. Symp., 1973; 4, 275.
25. Murdoch, G.; Hughes, J. in "Perspectives in Biomedical Engineering," Kenedi, R.M., ed., MacMillan Press Ltd., London, 1973, pp. 67-72.
26. Scott, R.N. in "Advances in Biomedical Engineering and Medical Physics," vol. 2, Levine, S.N., ed., Wiley-Interscience, New York, 1968, pp. 45-72.
27. Dagalakis, N.; Flink, J.; Stasikelis, P.; Burke, J.F.; Yannis, I.V., J. Biomed. Mater. Res., 1980; 14, 511.
28. Wang, P.Y.; Samji, N.A. in Ref. (2), pp. 29-37.
29. May, P.D. in Ref. (12), pp. 257-268.
30. Chvapil, M., J. Biomed. Mater. Res., 1977; 11, 721.
31. Braley, S.A. in Ref. (12), pp. 277-283.
32. Johnsson-Hegyeli, R. in Ref. (12), pp. 207-233.
33. Braley, S. in "Biomaterials," Stark, L.; Agarwal, G., eds., Plenum Publ., New York, 1969, pp. 67-89.
34. Myers, G.H.; Parsonnet, V., "Engineering in the Heart and Blood Vessels," Wiley-Interscience, New York, 1969, Chapt. 2-7.
35. Myers, G.H.; Parsonnet, V. in "Cardiac Engineering, Vol. 3 of Advances in Biomedical Engineering and Medical Physics," Nose, Y.; Levine, S.N., eds., Wiley-Interscience, New York, 1970, pp. 335-368.
36. Silver, M.D.; Datta, B.N.; Bowes, V.F., Arch. Pathol., March, 1975; 99, 132.
37. Lefrak, E.A.; Starr, A., "Cardiac Valve Prostheses," Appleton-Century-Crofts, New York, 1979.
38. Harasaki, H.; Snow, J.; Cloesmeyer, R.; Nose, Y., Inter. J. Artificial Organs, 1979; 2 (2), 73.
39. Bricker, D.L.; Beall, Jr., A.C.; DeBakey, M.E., Chest, 1970; 58, 566.
40. Vaughan, C.D.; Mattox, K.L.; Feliciano, D.V.; Beall, Jr., A.C.; DeBakey, M.E., J. Trauma, 1979; 19, 403.

41. Raithel, D.; Groitl, H. World J. Surgery, 1980; 4, 223.
42. Knutson, K.; Lyman, D.J. in Ref. (2), pp. 173-188.
43. Lyman, D.J.; Seifert, K.B.; Knowlton, H.; Albo, Jr., D., in Ref. (2), pp. 163-171.
44. Murabayashi, S.; Nose, Y. in Ref. (2), pp. 111-118.
45. Akutsu, T.; Yamamoto, N.; Serrato, M.A.; Denning, J.; Drummond, M.A. in Ref. (2), pp. 119-142.
46. Eskin, S.G.; Navarro, L.T.; Sybers, H.B.; O'Bannon, W.; DeBakey, M.E. in Ref. (2), pp. 43-161.
47. Pierce, W.S.; Brighton, J.A.; Donachy, J.H.; Landis, D.L.; Rosenberg, G.; Prophet, G.A.; White, W.J.; Waldhausen, J.A.; Arch. Surg. Chicago, 1970; 112, 1430.
48. Bregman, D.; Nichols, A.B.; Weiss, M.B.; Powers, E.R.; Martin, E.C.; Casarella, W.J., Am. J. Cardiol., 1980; 46, 261.
49. Santiago, J.V.; Clemens, A.H.; Clarke, W.L.; Kipnis, D.M., Diabetes, 1979; 28 (1), 71.
50. Gray, D.N. in Ref. (2), pp. 21-27.
51. Zapol, W.M.; Ketteringham, J. in Ref. (10), pp. 287-312.
52. Kulbe, K.D., Artificial Organs, 1979; 3, 143.
53. Kolff, W. in Ref. (10), pp. 1-28.
54. Kinney, S.E., Artificial Organs, 1979; 3, 379.
55. Langston, R.H.S., Artificial Organs, 1978; 2 (1), 55.
56. Sperling, T.D.; Bering, E.A.; Pollack, S.V.; Vaughan, H.G., eds., "Visual Prosthesis, The Interdisciplinary Dialogue," Academic Press, New York, 1971.

RECEIVED April 23, 1984

2

Synthetic Polymeric Biomaterials

ALLAN S. HOFFMAN

Department of Chemical Engineering and Center for Bioengineering, University of Washington, Seattle, WA 98105

> A review is presented of the applications of synthetic polymers in medicine. The major uses of these biomaterials are in devices and implants for diagnosis or therapy. The composition and properties, characterization, and biologic interactions of a wide variety of synthetic polymers are reviewed. Biologic testing and clearance of biomaterials for clinical use are also covered.

Biomaterials and Their Uses

There is a wide variety of materials which are foreign to the body and which are used in contact with body fluids. These include totally synthetic materials as well as reconstituted or specially treated human or animal tissues. Some are needed only for short term applications while others are, hopefully, useful for the lifetime of the individual. The various uses of such foreign materials, otherwise known as "biomaterials" may be generally categorized as devices or implants, for diagnosis or therapy. They include invasive instrumentation (e.g., catheters); implanted devices or instruments (e.g., pacemakers, hydrocephalus tubes); extra-corporeal devices in series with blood flow (e.g., artificial kidney, heart-lung blood oxygenators); implanted parts (or whole) of hard structural elements (e.g., hip joints, teeth); implanted parts (or whole) of organs (e.g., heart valves, heart assist devices, skin); and implanted soft tissue substitutes (e.g., blood vessels, tendon, ureter).

One may also list the "ideal" requirements for selecting a particular biomaterial for a particular end-use. The material chosen should have the required physical properties (as strength, elasticity, permeability); it must be easily purified, fabricated and sterilized; it should maintain the needed physical properties and function in vivo over the desired time period (1 hour, 1 day, 1 year, 10 years, patient lifetime); and it should not induce undesirable host reactions (as blood clotting, tissue necrosis,

0097-6156/84/0256-0013$06.00/0
© 1984 American Chemical Society

carcinogenesis, allergenic responses, etc.). It should be noted that very few (if any) biomaterials in fact conform to all these criteria. Nevertheless, a wide variety of biomaterials have emerged and are in daily use in the clinic. Table I identifies six classes of biomaterials, and the many different forms in which they are found in devices and implants. The first five classes are clearly separate types of materials, while the sixth class, "Composites," includes systems which combine different forms of materials within any one class (as a rubber diaphragm reinforced with a fabric) or different classes of materials (as a heart valve made of a metal and different synthetic polymers or of natural animal tissues and different synthetic polymers). This paper is a review of the field of synthetic polymeric biomaterials and as such will not attempt to cover natural tissue biomaterials, carbons, metals, or ceramics. A general reference list is provided which does cover all of these materials and their applications in medicine.

Table I. Classes and Forms of Biomaterials

CLASSES	FORMS

I. Polymers
  a) fibers
  b) rubbers
  c) plastics
	films or membranes
	fibers or fabrics
	tubes
	powders or particles
	molded shapes
	bags or containers, etc.
	liquids solids (adhesives)

II. Metals	cast or molded shapes powders or particles fibers
III. Ceramics	molded shapes powders or particles liquids solids (cements)
IV. Carbons	machined shapes coatings fibers
V. Natural Tissues	fibers natural forms also, reconstituted as films, tubes, fibers, etc.
VI. Composites	coatings fibrous felts or sheets fiber or fabric-reinforced shapes, etc.

Synthetic Polymeric Biomaterials

Synthetic polymers make up by far the broadest and most diverse class of biomaterials used. This is mainly because synthetic polymers are available with such a wide variety of compositions and properties and also because they may be fabricated readily into complex shapes and structures. In addition, their surfaces may be readily modified physically, chemically, or biochemically.

This wide variety of synthetic polymeric biomaterials can be seen in Figures 1-3, which are separated into categories of solid, liquid, or water-soluble polymer systems (Figure 1). The solid polymeric biomaterials may be subdivided into soft and/or rubbery materials, amorphous and hard materials, and semi-crystalline materials. Figure 2 shows examples in each of these categories for a wide variety of biomaterials applications.

Water sorption in biomaterials is very important to the functioning of some polymers, such as hydrogels in soft contact lenses. Water uptake may also lead to absorption of ions and other molecules, as enzymes, which can cause biodegradation of the polymer, especially if it contains susceptible bonds. Figure 3 lists the relative water sorption of a variety of polymeric biomaterials. Figure 4 indicates the most commonly encountered biodegradable repeating bond units in polymer backbones. Such polymers generally degrade via hydrolysis reactions. Biodegradability may or may not be desired in a polymeric implant.

An additional complication of polarity or polar additives in polymers is the possibility of extraction of polymer additives, smaller molecules, etc. into the surrounding biological fluids. This can lead to local or even systemic toxic responses (see below). Table II lists some potential extractables in polymers.

Table II. Some Potential Extractables in Commercial Polymers

- Catalyst fragments
- Anti-oxidants
- U.V. stabilizers
- Plasticizers
- Low molecular weight polymer molecules
- Surface active agents
  (lubricants, wetting agents, anti-static agents)
- Dyes
- Flame retardants
- Fragments of fillers, reinforcing agents
- Polymer degradation byproducts

Biologically Active Polymers

Reactable sites as -OH, -COOH, or $-NH_2$ may be present on the polymer backbone, or may be introduced via a free radical

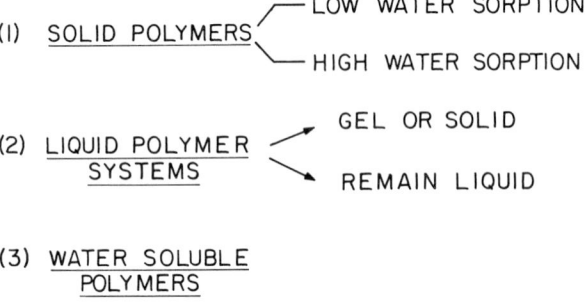

Figure 1. Polymeric biomaterials.

	PROPERTIES	EXAMPLES	USES
(a)	SOFT (RUBBERY)		
	—LOW WATER SORPTION	SR, PU, PVC	TUBES, DIAPHRAGMS, COATINGS, IMPLANTS, PACEMAKERS, ADHESIVES, BLOOD BAGS
	—HIGH WATER SORPTION	PHEMA	CONTACT LENS, BURN DRESSING, COATINGS
(b)	AMORPHOUS, HARD	PMMA	CONTACT LENS, IOL, DENTAL AND ORTHOPEDIC CEMENTS
(c)	SEMI-CRYSTALLINE		
	—LOW WATER SORPTION	PET, PP, PTFE	SUTURES, VASCULAR GRAFTS, SEWING ANCHORS, TISSUE INGROWTH
		NYLONS, PGA	SUTURES, (BIODEGRADABLE)
		PE	IUD, BONE JOINTS,
		PFEP	CATHETERS
		CA	HOLLOW FIBER DIALYSER, CONTACT LENS
	—MODERATE WATER SORPTION	CELL	DIALYSIS MEMBRANE

Figure 2. Solid polymeric biomaterials. Symbols used:
- SR   Silicone rubber (crosslinked)
- PU   Polyurethane rubber
- PVC   Poly(vinyl chloride)
- PHEMA Poly(hydroxyethyl methacrylate)
- PMMA Poly(methyl methacrylate)
- PET   Poly(ethylene terephthalate)
- PP   Polypropylene
- PTFE Poly(tetrafluoroethylene)
- PGA   Poly(glycolic acid)
- PE   Polyethylene
- PFEP Poly(perfluoro ethylene-propylene)
- CA   Cellulose acetate
- Cell Cellulose

	"NON-POLAR"	- - - - - - - -	"POLAR"	
"POLARITY"	NEGLIGIBLE	LOW	MED.	HIGH
WATER SORPTION	< 1% - - - - - -	1-5% - - -	5-15% - - -	>15% - - - -
EXAMPLES	PTFE PE PP	SR PET PMMA	PU	Nylon Cellulose PHEMA PAAm

Figure 3. Relative "polarity" (i.e., water sorption) of some solid polymeric biomaterials. (Additional symbol: PAAm = polyacrylamide.)

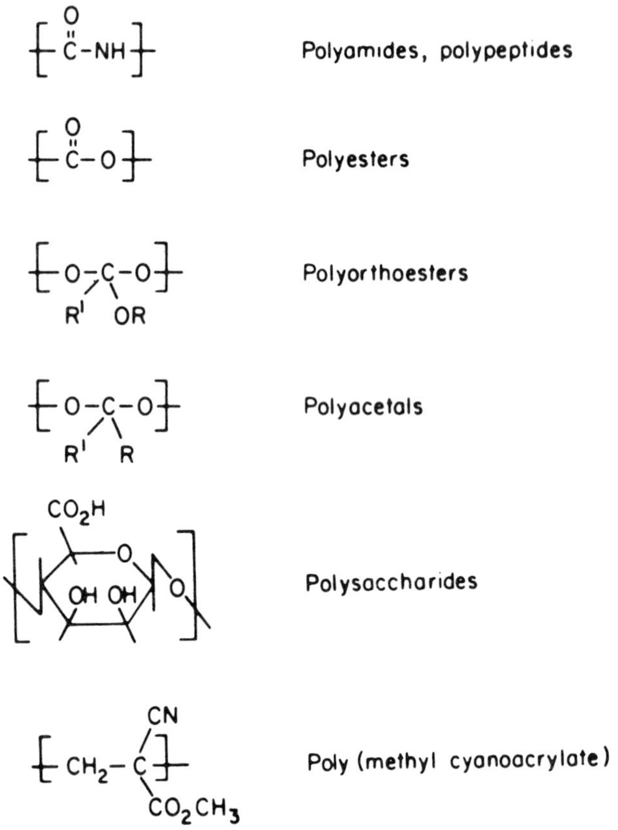

$-[-\overset{O}{\underset{\|}{C}}-NH-]-$ Polyamides, polypeptides

$-[-\overset{O}{\underset{\|}{C}}-O-]-$ Polyesters

$-[-O-\underset{R^I\ OR}{C}-O-]-$ Polyorthoesters

$-[-O-\underset{R^I\ R}{C}-O-]-$ Polyacetals

(cyclic sugar structure with CO$_2$H, OH, OH, O) Polysaccharides

$-[-CH_2-\underset{CO_2CH_3}{\overset{CN}{C}}-]-$ Poly(methyl cyanoacrylate)

Figure 4. Repeat units in some biodegradable polymer backbones.

graft polymerization reaction. Figure 5 lists the variety of process techniques which may be used to create macroradical sites for grafting polar monomers onto more inert polymer backbones. The presence of such groups on the surface of (or throughout) polymers can permit the chemical immobilization of a wide variety of biologically functional molecules (Table III). Such active compounds may also be electrostatically "bound" to the polymer by opposite charge or acid-base attractions, or they may be entrapped within the polymer.

Table III. Some Biologically Active Species which may be Immobilized on or within Polymeric Biomaterials

> Enzymes
> Antibodies
> Antigens
> Anti-thrombogenic agents
> Antibiotics
> Antibacterial agents
> Contraceptives
> Hormones
> Anticancer agents
> Drug antagonists
> Drug analogs
> Other drugs, in general
> Sugars and polysaccharides
> Cells

A wide variety of drug delivery systems has been developed for achieving a regulated or controlled release of therapeutic agents over a sustained and pre-determined period of time. Polymers may be utilized as diffusion-controlling barrier membranes (in "reservoir" devices), matrices for containment and release of active agents (in "monolithic" devices), or more simply as containers, conduits, or other components of the device. The polymers may be designed to resist attack or to erode or degrade. In particular, a number of biodegradable polymers have been specially synthesized for release of active agents inside the body, during or after which the polymer disappears as it erodes or degrades and is metabolized.

Another interesting new combination of polymers and biological species may be synthesized by covalently binding biologically active molecules to the surface of polymeric particles, such as those prepared in microemulsion polymerizations. Thus, if a particular antibody is attached, the microparticles will be attracted to specific antigenic sites in the body. If these sites are on specific cancer cells, and if an anti-cancer drug is incorporated into or onto the micro-article, with the possibility of subsequent release from the particle, then specific drugs may be delivered to specific sites in the

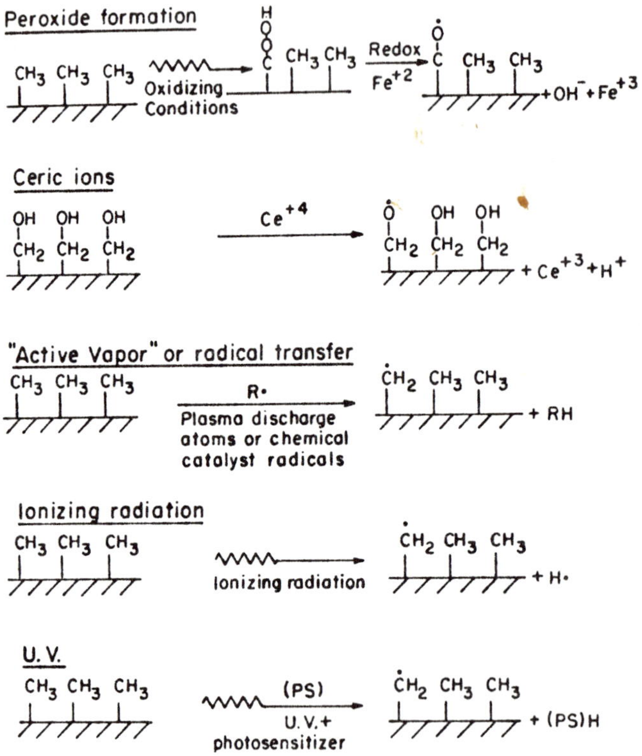

Figure 5. Examples of techniques and reactions for generating radicals on surfaces. (Note: The precise nature of the radical intermediates formed has not been elucidated in some cases. Representations in this figure show schematically radical species which might be formed.)

body, using the body's own circulatory system to transport the particles.

Cells may also be cultured within or on the outside of hollow fiber exchange devices and a patient's blood may be circulated through the device for treatment of various diseases (e.g., using pancreatic beta cells for diabetes patients in an "artificial pancreas," or using liver cells in an "artificial liver" during hepatic failure). Table IV lists some general examples of biomedical uses of immobilized biomolecule or cell systems.

Table IV. Some Examples of Uses of Immobilized Biomolecule or Cell Systems

Improved biocompatibility

Drug delivery

Cell "finders" and "markers" (via antibody-antigen binding)

Diagnostic kits

Enzyme reactors (including artificial organs)

Biomedical sensors or electrodes

The Polymer Biologic Interface

When a foreign surface is exposed to a biological environment, there is a natural tendency to destroy (digest) the foreign object or, failing that, to "wall it off" and cover (encapsulate) the object. The biologic species which are involved in this process are proteins and cells (Figure 6). The first event is generally to coat the polymer surface with a layer of proteins; the composition and organization of this layer will influence the subsequent cellular events (see below). Thus, it is essential that one characterize and reproduce the surface of the biomaterial to be used in any implant or device.

There are a number of other important factors which influence the biological interaction and ultimate fate of a biomaterial in the body. Biomaterial properties, such as purity, tendency to absorb water and degrade are clearly important. Also, the design of the device or implant, the flow of biological fluids by the foreign surfaces or movement of the implant within a tissue space, the test techniques selected to assay biomaterial responses in vitro or in vivo (in different animal species), and the implantation itself can all contribute to the ultimate fate of the implant device. Table V lists these factors and Table VI details important biomaterial surface properties.

Table V. Important Factors in Biomaterial-Biologic Interactions

  I. Biomaterial
     A. Bulk properties
     B. Surface properties
     C. Handling, packaging

  II. Biologic Environment
     A. In vitro vs. in vivo
     B. Species

  III. Physical Factors
     A. System design; flow characteristics
     B. Time, temperature
     C. Air interface

Table VI. Important Material and Surface Properties at the Biomaterial Interface

  I. Composition
     -- hydrophilic/hydrophobic
     -- polar/apolar
     -- high energy/low energy
     -- wettable/non-wettable
     -- acid/base
     -- anionic/cationic
     -- uniform/domain structure

  II. Sorbed Water
     -- oriented
     -- structured
     -- "free"

  III. "Compliance"
     -- flexibility of chain ends, loops
     -- glass trainsition

  IV. Roughness
     -- scale and intensity
     -- porosity
     -- local imperfections
     -- gas nuclei

Over the past several years, a great deal of effort has gone into characterizing the biomaterial surface composition. Contact angle measurements, infra-red reflectance spectroscopy (MIRS, FTIR), and electron microscopy (XPS or ESCA) have been the most popular techniques utilized. ESCA has become a very useful tool, since it yields an average composition of the top 10-100 Å of the biomaterial surface (although the measurement is made at low temperature and under high vacuum). The surface topography is also very important, particularly when compared to the scale of proteins and cells (Figures 7, 8). Surface roughness has been visualized using optical and (especially) scanning electron microscopy. Profilometry has occasionally been used. Table VII lists various common biomaterials in approximate categories of increasing roughness.

Table VII. Relative Roughness of Some Biomaterials

Very Smooth:	Pyrolitic Carbons; Metals
Smooth:	Silicone Rubbers; Polyurethanes; Polyethylene; Polyvinylchloride
Microrough:	Grafted Polyethylenes; Micro-porous materials (as PTFE)
Medium Rough:	Woven Dacron, Teflon fabrics; Medium porosity materials
Very Rough:	Knitted, velour or non-woven fabrics; macro-porous materials; sand-blasted materials

Biologic Responses

One may imagine that the body is divided into two systems: (1) the soft tissues, surfaces and spaces, organs and nerves, external to cardiovascular system (called the extravascular system); and (2) the cardiovascular-blood system (called the intravascular system).

Tissue responses. The major response to foreign bodies in the extravascular system is the inflammatory process. Whether the foreign "body" is a molecule or a solid particle or object, there is inflammation in the vicinity and the proteins and cells attempt to digest the foreign element and convert it to tolerable metabolites. Most foreign devices or implants are not readily or rapidly metabolized and the alternate fate is to be encapsulated in a fibrous collagen scar tissue capsule. If the biomaterial is porous, this tissue may be deposited within the pores, and such a process may be useful in anchoring and/or plugging the implant. Indeed, some researchers have attempted to develop porous implants (as a fibrous vessel prosthesis) which would

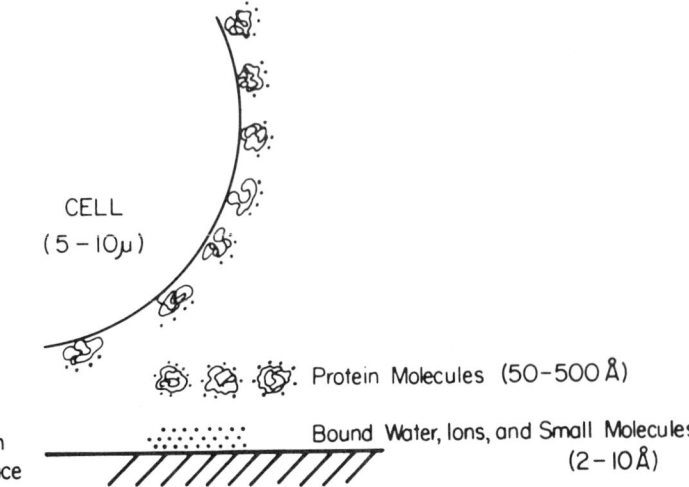

Figure 6. The primary interactions at a foreign biomaterial interface in the body are first with proteins and then with living cells. The drawing is schematic, and not to scale.

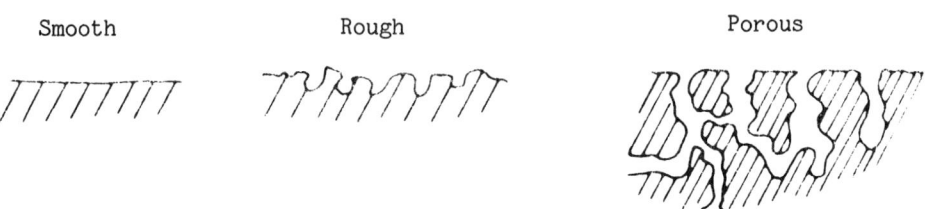

Figure 7. Biomaterial surfaces may be "smooth," "rough," or "porous" (schematic).

permit the reconstruction of the tissue being replaced while the implant itself slowly degrades and disappears.

In some cases the material may evolve toxic substances, and cause tissue necrosis (the question of carcinogenesis is considered below), or it may be of a specific geometry (as asbestos fibers) to induce excessive collagen fibrosis, which can be undesirable. Figure 9 summarizes these responses.

Blood responses. Blood is the fluid which transports body nutrients and waste products to and from the extravscular tissue and organs, and as such is a vital and special body tissue. The major response of blood to any foreign surface (which includes most extravascular surfaces of the body's own tissues) is first to deposit a layer of proteins and then, within seconds to minutes, a thrombus composed of blood cells and fibrin (a fibrous protein). The character of the thrombus will depend on the rate and pattern of blood flow in the vicinity. Thus, the design of the biomaterial system is particularly important for cardiovascular implants and devices. The thrombus may break off and flow downstream as an embolus and this can be a very dangerous event. In some cases the biomaterial interface may eventually "heal" and become covered with a "passive" layer of protein and/or cells. Growth of a continuous monolayer of endothelial cells onto this interface is the one most desirable end-point for a biomaterial in contact with blood. Figure 10 summarizes possible blood responses to polymeric biomaterials.

Testing and Clearance of Polymeric Biomaterials

Test techniques for both tissue and blood responses of biomaterials have evolved significantly over the past several years. Increased government regulation of biomaterials in medical devices (as legislated in the U.S.A. in 1976 by the Medical Devices Amendments Act) has stimulated the development of a number of common in vitro and in vivo animal test systems for screening a wide variety of biomaterials and devices or implants for both tissue and blood responses. Tissue tests encompass a variety of in vitro and in vivo techniques. Blood tests include in vitro, ex vivo, and in vivo techniques. It is unlikely that successful medical devices or implants can be perfected for human use without such preliminary in vitro and (especially) animal tests.

Ultimately, the biomaterial device or implant system must be tested clinically, first in small scale studies, then later, if all goes well, in larger multi-center clinical trials. The FDA, the device or implant manufacturer and their "monitor" (who will interface with the physician), the physician ("investigator") and his institutional review board, and finally the patient are all involved in responsible roles in the clinical trials, the clearance process, and the eventual general clinical use.

Smooth
Rough
Porous
Rounded-up cells vs. Spread Cells

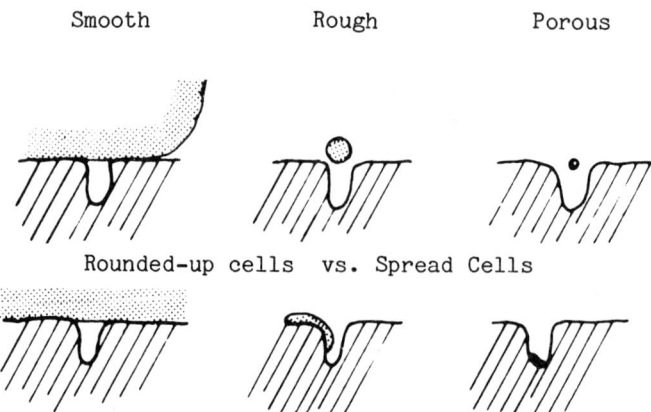

Figure 8. The importance of the scale and intensity of biomaterial surface "roughness" will depend upon the relative size and interaction of cells on that surface (schematic).

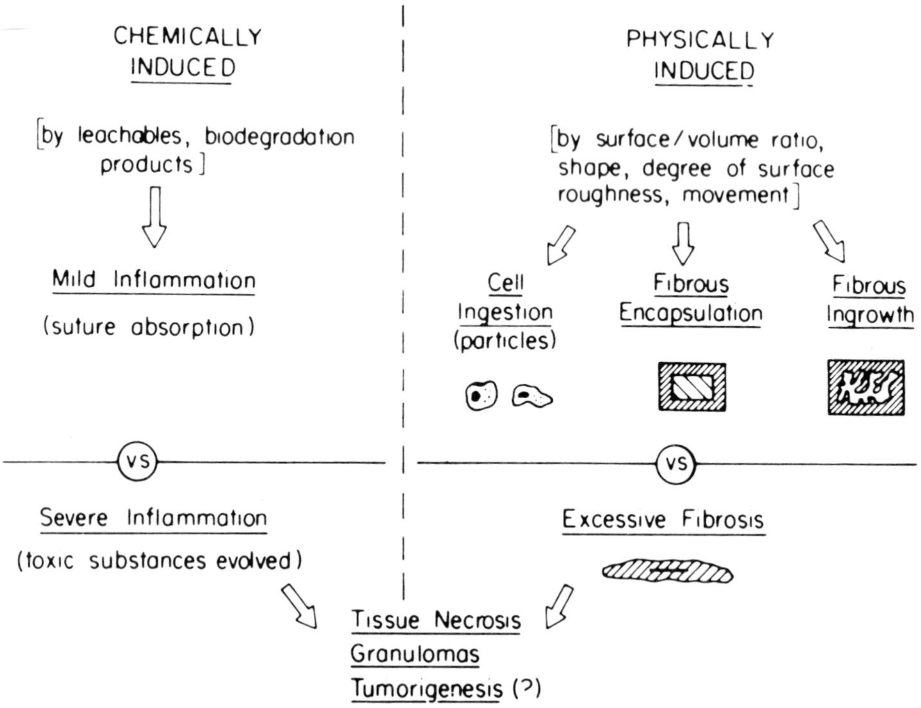

CHEMICALLY INDUCED
[by leachables, biodegradation products]
Mild Inflammation
(suture absorption)
PHYSICALLY INDUCED
[by surface/volume ratio, shape, degree of surface roughness, movement]
Cell Ingestion (particles)
Fibrous Encapsulation
Fibrous Ingrowth
VS
VS
Severe Inflammation
(toxic substances evolved)
Excessive Fibrosis
Tissue Necrosis
Granulomas
Tumorigenesis (?)

Figure 9. Tissue responses to foreign materials in the extravascular space. The overall process involved in all cases is called the inflammatory process.

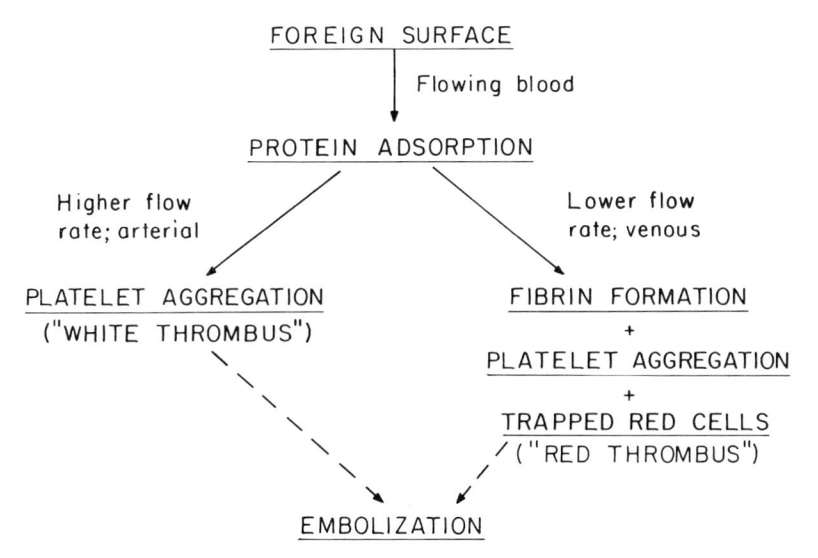

```
                    FOREIGN SURFACE
                           │ Flowing blood
                           ▼
                    PROTEIN ADSORPTION
      Higher flow       ╱              ╲      Lower flow
      rate; arterial   ╱                ╲     rate; venous
                      ▼                  ▼
            PLATELET AGGREGATION       FIBRIN FORMATION
             ("WHITE THROMBUS")               +
                       ╲              PLATELET AGGREGATION
                        ╲                     +
                         ╲            TRAPPED RED CELLS
                          ╲          ╱  ("RED THROMBUS")
                           ▼        ▼
                          EMBOLIZATION
```

Figure 10. Blood responses to foreign materials depend on the material as well as its design and the character of the blood flow near the biomaterial surface.

Finally, something should be said about the possibility of biomaterial-induced carcinogenesis in humans. In the absence of evolution of chemical carcinogens by the foreign material, there is no evidence for carcinogenesis in humans caused by the biomaterials currently used in implants or devices. This is in contrast to the tumorigenic responses of rodents to many of these same biomaterials. If the latent period for foreign body tumorigenesis in humans is merely much longer than that in rodents, sufficient time may not have elapsed to conclude that tumors induced by implanted biomaterials will not eventually be seen in humans. On the other hand, it is even more likely that this latent period -- if it exists -- would be longer than the useful lifespan of the implant.

Literature Cited

Polymeric Biomaterials
1. Cooper, S.L.; Hoffman, A.S.; Peppas, N.A.; Ratner, B.D., Eds.; "Morphology, Structure, and Interactions of Biomaterials"; ADVANCES IN CHEMISTRY SERIES, American Chemical Society: Washington, D.C., 1982.
2. Hoffman, A.S. J. Appl. Polymer Sci., Appl. Polymer Symp. 1977, 31, 313.
3. Major biomaterials journals or annual publications: J. Biomed. Matls. Res. (Wiley); Biomatls., Med. Devices, Artif. Org. (M. Dekker); Biomaterials (IPC Sci. and Tech. Press); Trans. Soc. for Biomatls. (Soc. for Biomaterials)
4. Kronenthal, R.L.; Oser, Z.; Martin, E., Eds.; "Polymers in Medicine and Surgery"; POLYMER SCIENCE AND TECHNOLOGY Vol. 8, Plenum Press: New York, 1975.
5. Park, J.B. "Biomaterials: An Introduction"; Plenum: New York, 1979.
6. Ratner, B.D.; Hoffman, A.S., in "Hydrogels for Medical and Related Applications"; Andrade, J.D., Ed.; ACS SYMPOSIUM SERIES No. 31, American Chemical Society: Washington, D.C., 1976; pp. 1-36.
7. Sedlacek, B.; Overberger, C.G.; Mark, H., Eds.; "Medical Polymers: Chemical Problems"; POLYMER SYMPOSIUM No. 66, Interscience-Wiley: New York, 1979.
8. Szycher, M.; Robinson, W.J., Eds.; "Synthetic Biomedical Polymers: Concepts and Applications"; Technomic Publ. Co.: Westport, CT, 1980.
9. Winter, G.; Gibbons, D.; Plenk, H., Eds. Proc. 1st World Congress on Biomaterials, Wiley: London, 1981.

Implants and Devices
10. Akutsu, T. "Artificial Heart: Total Replacement and Partial Support"; Excerpta Medica: Amsterdam, 1975.
11. Baker, R.W.; Lonsdale, H.K. Chem. Tech. 1975, 5, 668.
12. Chang, T.M.S. "Artificial Cells"; C.C. Thomas: Springfield, IL, 1972.

13. Major journals or annual publications: Trans. Amer. Soc. Artif. Int. Org. (ASAIO); Artif. Org. (ISAO); J. Artificial Org. (Wichtig); Proceedings of the Devices and Technology Branch, Contractors Meeting 1979, NHLBI, NIH, U.S. Dept. of H.H.S., Publ. No. 81-2022, November 1980.
14. Kolff, W.J. "Artificial Organs"; Wiley: New York, 1976.
15. Kolff, W.J. Artif. Org. 1977, 1, 8.
16. Tanquary, A.C.; Lacey, R.E., Eds.; "Controlled Release of Biologically Active Agents"; ADVANCES IN EXPERIMENTAL MEDICINE AND BIOLOGY Vol. 47, Plenum: New York, 1976.

Modification and Characterization of Biomaterials

17. Guidelines for Physicochemical Characterization of Biomaterials, Devices and Technology Branch, NHLBI, NIH, U.S. Dept. of H.H.S., Publ. No. 80-2186, September 1980.
18. Hoffman, A.S., in "Science and Technology of Polymer Processing," Suh, N.P.; Sung, N.H., Eds.; MIT Press: Cambridge, MA, 1979; p. 200.
19. Hoffman, A.S., in "Biomedical Polymers"; Dusek, K., Ed.; ADVANCES IN POLYMER SCIENCE special volume, Springer-Verlag: Berlin, to be published in 1983-84.
20. Rembaum, A.S.; Yen, S.P.S.; Molday, R.S. J. Macromol. Sci. Chem. 1979, A13, 603.

Biologic Responses, Testing and Clearance of Polymeric Biomaterials

21. Bruck, S.C., "Properties of Biomaterials in the Physiologic Environment"; CRC Press: Boca Raton, FL, 1980.
22. Dobelle, W.H.; Morton, W.A.; Lysaght, M.J.; Burton, E.M. Artif. Org. 1980, 4, 1.
23. Everything You Always Wanted to Know about the Medical Device Amendments and Weren't Afraid to Ask, U.S. Dept. of H.H.S., FDA, 8757 Georgia Ave., Silver Spring, MD 20910, Publ. No. FDA-77-5006, 1977.
24. Guidelines for Blood-Material Interactions, Devices and Technology Branch, NHLBI, NIH, U.S. Dept. of H.H.S., Publ. No. 80-2185, September 1980.
25. Vroman, L.; Leonard, E.F., Eds.; "The Behavior of Blood and its Components at Interfaces"; ANNALS OF N.Y. ACADEMY OF SCIENCE, No. 283, 1977.
26. Williams, D.F., Ed.; "Fundamental Aspects of Biocompatibility"; Vols. I and II; CRC Press: Boca Raton, FL, 1981.

RECEIVED March 19, 1984

Artificial Organs and the Immune Response

P. Y. WANG and C. CHAMBERS

Laboratory of Chemical Biology, Institute of Biomedical Engineering & Department of Physiology, Faculty of Medicine, University of Toronto, Ontario, Canada M5S 1A8

> Availability and immunological limitations of homografts have stimulated the development of artificial organs. Many extracorporeal and implantable devices have achieved remarkable success in substituting defective natural functions. Recently, interests in developing controlled release delivery systems to mimic the functions of the endocrines, e.g., in contraceptive steroid delivery, may extend this area of biotechnology to affect a large number of healthy individuals. Possible immune responses to synthetic materials used in fabrication should be among important aspects of artificial organ research. Antigenicity can be assessed by many antibody detection methods. The radioimmunoassay method is particularly suitable and our results show that C57BL/6 mice are high responders to many water-soluble biomedical polymers of acrylic acid, acrylamide, vinylpyrrolidone, vinyl alcohol, Na^+ styrenesulfonate, etc. Others have observed that some of these polyanions can influence the outcome of the immune response. Insoluble polymers are not as easily assessed, but an indirect method has shown that several inert inorganic and organic biomedical polymers can also alter the immune response. The scanty information available at present already indicates that artificial organs may not be immune to responses from the immune system.

Advances in modern medical practice have increased the use of plastic materials for tissue or organ replacements as well as

0097-6156/84/0256-0031$06.00/0
© 1984 American Chemical Society

in devices which may help to restore the physiological state of the body. Prior to use, the suitability of a material for biomedical applications must be established. Often, the material performance is assessed by measuring the physical, chemical, and biocompatibility properties. Since they do not occur in nature, many synthetic polymers are believed to generate no immune response. There is sufficient information available at present to indicate that an immune response can indeed be induced by some polymer components in drug formulations or in surgical implants. This paper briefly surveys the immunological events from presently rather limited amount of available data in this developing area of biomaterials research.

Historical Background (1)

The early study of the immune response evolved mostly from clinical observation of infectious diseases. The "resistance" to a second infection of the same disease was noted around 500 B.C. An early form of vaccine was the rather unsafe use of live smallpox organisms given to people for protection against infection. Later, Jenner vaccinated against smallpox with the non-virulent cowpox organism. However, it was not until the late 19th century that the role of antibodies in the defense against infection became gradually apparent. Soon, the presence of a substance in the serum that could combine with red blood cells in vitro and made the cells resistant to the ricin toxin was observed by Ehrlich. The observation was the first evidence of antigen-antibody complexing which was part of the defense mechanism. This led to further studies of antigen (abbrev. as Ag) immunochemistry, and the immunology of antibody (abbrev. as Ab) production, particularly with proteins, plant and bacterial products. With the discovery of the ABO types in human blood group substances by Lansteiner, the genetic control of the immune system was also realized.

Concepts of the Immune System (1, 2)

The adaptive or acquired immune system in mammals is characterized by three features, i.e., specificity, recognition, and memory. These features depend on the intrinsic ability of the lymphocytes to recognize a substance as foreign, and allow an increased efficiency of response upon a second exposure to the same substance. An Ag is a material capable of reacting specifically with the Ab produced as a manifestation of the response. It is also possible for an Ag, especially in high doses, to produce a state of non-responsiveness referred to as tolerance. For an Ag to induce a response, it should have a relatively large molecular weight, e.g., greater than 1,000 daltons. Otherwise, it is referred to as a hapten which would not induce a response by itself, unless linked to a polymeric "carrier" such as poly- (vinyl alcohol), poly- acrylamide, etc. The immune response produced is affected by the presentation of the Ag to the host, e.g., the state of the Ag, adjuvant, dose, route, etc., as well as by genetic factors. The primary effectors of the immune system are the lymphocytes, and their precursors are the stem cells in the bone marrow. One sub-population of the stem cells differentiates in the thymus (i.e. the T-cells), while the other matures primarily in the bone marrow and the gut-associated lymphoid tissues (i.e. the B-cells). Accordingly, there are two types of responses depending on the cell sub-population that is activated. The first is the cell mediated response, if the T-lymphocytes are stimulated. The other is the humoral response, if only the B-cells are involved. However, most B-cells which respond by releasing Ab also may require a T-cell "helper" signal to transform and proliferate into plasma cells. This series of events is further complicated by the regulation of such responses which involve T-suppressor cells, participation of macrophages, other accessory cells, negative feedback from the Ab themselves, genetic controls, and possibly other factors yet to be delineated.

Antibody Detection Methods (3)

There are many well-established methods for the detection of immune responses, especially when the Ab are released into the systemic circulation. Earlier, the agglutination of bacteria was used to show the presence of specific Ab in serum of infected individuals. The formation of Ag-Ab complex can also be observed as aggregates in the ring test, precipitin reaction or various gel media. More recently, sensitive methods are developed to detect Ab in the ug to pg range. Details of the hemagglutination, hemolysis, radioimmunoassay (abbrev. as RIA) and plaque forming assay, etc., can be found in a standard manual (3). The limits of sensitivity of these methods are shown in Table I. However, all these Ab analyses are devised to study natural or haptenic Ag, and may not always be applicable to the detection of Ag-Ab interaction involving highly water-soluble non-biological polymers that are strong polyelectrolytes. Thus, adaption and use of these classical methods to the synthetic polymers should be made with caution.

Experimental

Several mouse strains were observed to produce Ab after stimulation with water-soluble synthetic polymers (4). The C57BL/6 strain was found to be most responsive. Therefore, in this study several common water-soluble polymer Ag were used to

Table I. Analytical Sensitivity of Some Detection
Methods for Ab

Methods	Sensitivity (μg Ab/ml serum)
Precipitation	20
Gel Diffusion	3 to 200
Hemagglutination	0.001 to 1
Hemolysis	0.0001 to 0.01
Complement Fixation	0.1
RIA	0.001

induce Ab production in groups of five C57BL/6 mice for each experiment. The polymer Ag were emulsified in Freund's complete adjuvant, and injected intraperitoneally as described previously (4). At regular intervals, the rodents were bled and the sera were separated from the coagulated cellular components (4). Presence of Ab in the sera was detected by the solid phase RIA. Briefly, 50 μl aliquots of a specific Ag solution containing 2% bovine serum albumin (abbrev. as BSA) were added to a number of the 96-well plastic assay plate which was then incubated for 2 hr at 37°C to allow the Ag to become adsorbed onto the plastic. The Ag-coated wells were washed 3x with a BSA-containing buffer, and 50 μl aliquots of a serially diluted Ab solution were added accordingly to the coated wells. After 2 hr at room temperature for Ab interaction with the adsorbed Ag, the wells were again washed, and then treated with 50 μl aliquots of an ^{125}I-labelled rabbit anti-mouse Ab fragment. The plate was incubated at 4°C for 16 hr, and the wells were washed once more. After cutting the wells apart, the levels of gamma-ray emitted by each sample were counted, and the results were reported as the maximum in geometric serial dilutions of the anti-serum that showed Ab activity after deduction of any background activities from the control which had normal mouse serum in place of the Ab solution.

Results

Several readily available biomedical polymers (Table II) were used as Ag to induce immune response in C57BL/6 mice and the Ab in the sera were detected by RIA. The results in Table II show that under the present experimental conditions, PVA, PAA, and

PAM are weakly or moderately immunogenic, while PSS and PVP are more potent Ag comparable to some natural Ag. Typically, the more immunogenic PSS exhibits a dose-response relationship (Table III). Doses as low as 10^{-3} µg can induce detectable Ab by the RIA, but almost a million-fold increase in the immunizing dose of PSS is required in order to obtain a substantially higher Ab titre, and the optimal response decreases rather rapidly (Table III). An apparent secondary response is observed when the mice were immunized with a sub-optimal dose followed by a booster injection (Table IV). This secondary response decreased to a lower level of Ab titre in about 1 week. Similarly, PVP is also known to induce such responses in mice (5).

Table II. Antigenic Biomedical Polymers Tested in C57BL/6 Mice

Abbrev. Names[a]	Max. RIA Ab Titre (2^n dilutions)
PSS	4096
PVP	4096
PVA	64
PAA	1024
PAM	16[b]

[a]PSS: Poly(styrenesulfonate Na$^+$); PVP: Poly(vinylpyrrolidone); PVA: poly(vinyl alcohol); PAA: Poly(acrylic acid); PAM: Poly(acrylamide).
[b]Detected by hemagglutination assay; immune serum from SJL mice.

Table III. Dose-Response Relationship for PSS in C57BL/6 Mice

Dose (µg)	Max. RIA Ab Tire (2^n dilutions)
10^{-3}	256
10^{-2}	256
10^{-1}	256
10^2	256
5×10^2	1024
8×10^2	512
10^3	4096
5×10^3	512

Table IV. Responses to Two Injections of 0.1 µg PSS in C57BL/6 Mice

Days	RIA Ab Titre (2^n dilutions)
0 (1st Inj.)	–
10	128
15	256
28	32
35	16
38 (2nd Inj.)	–
42	1024
50	256
58	256
66	16

Discussion

In our previous report (4, 5), the antigenicity of some of the biomedical polymers shown in Table II has been evaluated by using hemagglutination as the Ab detection method. However, probably because of the chemical or physical characteristics of these synthetic polymers, this method does not always produce predictable results. The solid phase RIA has corrected this inconsistency, and most of the Ab titres shown in Table II to IV are reproducible to within $2^{n\pm 2}$ dilutions which are in the range of variation for this type of experiments. Therefore, synthetic polymers, some as shown in Table II at least, are not necessarily inactive to the immune system.

Although there are substantial amount of data available on responses to synthetic poly(amino acids) which are essentially pseudo-biological polymers, a survey of literatures has provided information mostly on PVP. For example, Andersson and coworkers (6) have shown that PVP can induce Ab production in adult thymectomized mice after irradiation, followed by reconstitution with B-cells isolated from the spleens of other non-treated mice with the same genetic background. Their experiment demonstrates that PVP is a T-independent Ag (4). Further studies have shown that such response in reconstituted mice is affected by the maturity of the B-cells, and in younger animals, the co-operation of T-cells is required (7). In addition, others have observed that low doses of PVP may stimulate a sub-population of T-cells (the helper cells) to enhance the Ab production by B-cells (8). The opposite effect occurs when higher or the optimal dose is given (9). There are also reports indicating that poly(acrylic acid) can be used to replace the helper cell functions aforementioned in the response to the T-dependent bacterial lipopolysaccharides (10).

For many water-insoluble polymers the immune response, if any, is more difficult to evaluate. Recently, Habal and coworkers (11) have reported a method to assess the effect of solid implant materials such as silicone, segmented polyether-polyurethane, poly(methyl methacrylate), and Bioglas using tumor-bearing mice as the experimental model. They have found that the B-cells from the test animals showed a reduced capacity for proliferation when stimulated by mitogens as compared to the controls. The results demonstrate once again that even the relatively biocompatible solid polymers may have a measurable effect on the immune system.

Besides the many immunological events that can be initiated by the synthetic polymers as just described, there are also the pathological implications to be considered, such as the in vivo fate of the Ag-Ab complexes. Consequently, there is an urgent need for emphasis on immunological studies of biomaterials. Meanwhile, from our data and the information in the literature as just described, it appears that artificial organs may not be immune to immune responses. But the long-term effects of such responses as well as these effects on the complement system seem to be much more complex than are realized at present.

Literature Cited

1. Roitt, I. "Essential Immunology"; Blackwell Scientific: London, 1980; p. 4.
2. Raff, M.C. Scientif. Amer. 1976, 234, 30.
3. Mishell, B.B.; Shiigi, S.M. "Selected Methods in Cellular Immunology"; W.H. Freeman: San Francisco, 1980.
4. Wang, P.Y. Advan. Biomaterials 1982, 3, 799.
5. Wang. P.Y.; Alouf, A.; Samji, N.; Wolinsky, S. Immunology '80 (4th Internat'l. Congr. Immunology, Internat'l. Union Immunol.) 17.4.21.
6. Andersson, B.; Blomgren, H. Cell. Immunol. 1971, 2, 411.
7. Andersson, B.; Blomgren. H. Nature 1975, 253, 476.
8. Braley-Mullen, H.; Lite, H. Develop. Immunol. 1981, 15, 401.
9. Inaba, K.; Nakano, K.; Muramatsu, S. Cell. Immunol. 1978, 39, 260.
10. Sjoberg, O.; Andersson, J.; Moller, G. Eur. J. Immunol. 1972, 2, 326.
11. Habal, M.B.; Powell, M.L.; Schimpff, R.D. J. Biomed. Mater. Res. 1980, 14, 455.

RECEIVED March 19, 1984

The Basics of Biomedical Polymers: Interfacial Factors

ROBERT E. BAIER

Advanced Technology Center, Calspan Corporation, Buffalo, NY 14225

Interfacial phenomena, including initial adsorption of macromolecular films, attachment of cells, and triggering of cellular aggregation and exudation, often dictate the suitability of materials for biomedical applications. These factors can be better understood, controlled and predicted if the chemistry of the interfacing materials is well characterized in advance. This is particularly true in implant environments where application of such diagnostic tools as internal reflection spectroscopy, contact angle checks, film thickness determinations, and surface electrical potential measurements can aid considerably in selecting materials for prosthetic devices that promote good tissue incorporation while remaining passive to blood elements. The predictive patterns developed serve well across a large span of bioadhesive problems from those in tissue and blood to those in saliva and the sea. Specific application of the concept of critical surface tension has led to significant success in the design and clinical acceptance of new human arterial grafts, and is aiding in the development of artificial hearts, and subperiosteal dental implants. With these data in hand, materials deficiencies become less of a limiting factor in biomedical device construction. A significant research need is for specification of the mechanical shear forces that are required to assure reliable detachment of even weakly bound biofouling films from the least adherent substrata now available.

0097-6156/84/0256-0039$06.00/0
© 1984 American Chemical Society

Interfacial phenomena often dictate the suitability of biomaterials for _in vivo_ use. In particular, the surface characteristics of various implants control the relative adhesive strengths obtained between biomaterials and the living tissues they touch. While great adhesive strength and immobility are desired for orthopedic and dental implants, minimal bioadhesion is critical to preventing thrombus formation in cardiovascular devices, or plaque buildup on oral prostheses. This overview addresses the principles of surface phenomena in biological environments, describes useful methods for sensitive analysis of the earliest interfacial events, and provides illustrations of their use for characterizing materials placed in the human body.

Scope of the Problem

Attention is directed to bioadhesive phenomena in the oral environment that present improved surface conditioning methods to promote excellent bonding between tissue and implanted prosthetic devices (1). Other important surface phenomena include those necessary to the safe and effective function of cardiovascular appliances such as the artificial heart and substitute blood vessels (2,3). Impressive similarities exist with biological fouling of materials in the sea (4). The primary interfacial events in these diverse systems--all wet, salty, and biochemically active--are similar enough to suggest that Nature has been most conservative in accommodating encounters with strange boundaries.

Research Premise

A major difficulty in many prior studies of biomedical implants in the dental, orthopedic, or cardiovascular environment, has been the tendency to focus on long term behavior of the materials-- from weeks to months to years post-implantation. There has seldom been proper implant characterization or even knowledge of their surface states at the time of placement or of the early bioadhesive sequelae (within minutes, hours and days) changing the surface properties to others that can promote or inhibit adhesion of formed biological elements (such as tissue cells or bacterial organisms) (5). In more traditional engineering studies, for example those dealing with the rate of biological fouling of heat exchange materials (as in power plant condenser tubes) and its consequences, an analogous ignorance of the initiating events has been commonly dismissed with the label "induction period." (6) In such engineering systems, as with biomedical implants, significant gains in our understanding of the performance and control of the devices is highly dependent upon better knowledge of the actual, initial microfouling events. The first adhesive layers prepare the devices for grosser biofouling, with consequent deterioration, functional losses, and degraded performance.

Improved Methods for Analysis of Interfacial Factors

Test plates allowing sensitive inspection of the first organic layers accumulating on their faces are among the more useful tools of the interfacial scientist interested in bioadhesive phenomena. In relevant biological locations and during actual use, these are most valuable in characterizing the first adsorbed or adherent layers. The primary technique permitting inspection of the "interface conversion layers" spontaneously adsorbed to all known materials exposed to the environments of the month, tissue (whether in living animal or human hosts or in culture in laboratory containers), blood, or the sea, is known as internal reflection infrared spectroscopy (7). In essence, the technique places the analyst inside the test material that serves as a "light pipe" for probing beams of electromagnetic energy. The spectroscopic "fingerprint" of the material first adsorbing at the plate surface may be recorded during the primary adhesive phase (8).

Such test plates have been incubated in the mouths of human volunteers (9) and similar studies have been completed in broths consisting of nutrient medium inoculated with specific microorganisms originally taken by micromanipulation techniques from the adherent plaque of human teeth (10). The plates obviously experience different events on their faces, dictated by specific surface property differences. Some plates emerge from the plaque forming challenge as clean and shiny as upon first immersion. Others accumulate typical dental "brown stains" from microbial colonizing films (11). Metallic test plates such as germanium or silicon are often used because their conductive properties prevent electric charge accumulation during scanning electron microscopic inspection. This eliminates the need for additional metallic overcoatings usually applied to SEM samples prior to microscopic viewing. Absence of the uniformly electron-dense metallic overcoat on the intrinsically organic conditioning films (and attached cellular layers) then allows the relative thicknesses and locations of the organic masses to be distinguished by the differences in their ability to suppress secondary electron emission--the process that provides the image of the common scanning electron micrograph--of the high-electron-density metallic substrata.

The test plates can be made in almost any shape and size, and placed in special intraoral holders worn in mouths of human volunteers. Such holders provide means to analyze the "skin" on one's teeth, the pellicle acquired by specific adsorption of salivary components before any successful colonization by microbial flora is noted (12).

Infrared spectral traces obtained by the internal reflection method applied through test plates exposed for only a few moments in the human mouth, demonstrate the presence of rapidly adsorbed proteinaceous matter. Thus, the reality of the "skin" on one's teeth, or on any other object immersed even momentarily in this rich biological environment, can be documented. It is made of the same substance--protein--that other natural "skins" are made of. The spectra reveal that the protein present in the acquired pellicles is glycoprotein in the main.

In addition to the internal reflection spectroscopic technique, there is a host of supporting methods. They range from techniques that estimate precise film thickness and refractive index to techniques that measure surface electrical property and wettability changes that are associated with protein film deposition (13).

Use of these nondestructive methods, applied sequentially and routinely to test materials exposed in biological environments of concern, has been illustrated previously in studies of the fouling of food processing equipment (14).

Typical Results

Simple modification of the surface chemistry of immersed solid materials, specifically to provide low surface energy ranges as indicated by critical surface tensions between 20 and 30 dynes/cm, prevents permanent interface conversion by spontaneously adsorbing glycoproteinaceous macromolecules. This induction of a poor "primer coat" inhibits the adhesion of biological cells; even those elements such as blood platelets specialized for the purpose of surface colonization are prevented from getting a successful "grip" on the substrata. Conversely, upward adjustment of a material's surface energy promotes stronger biological interactions (15).

With knowledge of the zones of surface energy that either favor or minimize adhesion in biological environments, it is now possible to design and develop improved prosthetic materials for a number of important applications.

Elsewhere, we have reviewed many of the areas of current research in bioadhesive phenomena: dental restoratives, prosthetic implants, surgical adhesives, and even improved coatings for the prevention of marine fouling on commercial ships (16).

Literature Cited

1. Natiella, J.R., Meenaghan, M.A., Flynn, H.E., Carter, J.M., Baier, R.E., and Akers, C.K., Unilateral Superiosteal Implants in Primates, Journal of Prosthetic Dentistry, 48:68-77, 1982.

2. Baier, R.E., The Organization of Blood Components Near Interfaces, Annals of the New York Academy of Sciences, 283:17-36, 1977.

3. Baier, R. E., Akers, C. K., Natiella, J. R., Meenaghan, M.A., and Wirth, J., Physiochemical Properties of Stabilized Umbilical Vein, Vascular Surgery, 14:145-157, 1980.

4. Goupil, D.W., DePalma, V.A., and Baier, R.E., Physical/Chemical Characteristics of the Macromolecular Conditioning Film in Biological Fouling, Proceedings of the Fifth International Congress on Marine Corrosion and Fouling, Graficas Orbe, S.L., Padill, 82, Madrid, Spain, pp 401-410, 1980.

5. Baier, R.E., Surface Properties Influencing Biological Adheaion, Chapt. 2 in Adhesion in Biological Systems (R.S. Manly, ed.), Academic Press, NY pp 15-48, 1970.

6. DePalma, V.A. and Baier, R.E., Microfouling of Metallic and Coated Metallic Flow Surfaces in Model Heat Exchange Cells, Proceedings of the Ocean Thermal Energy Conversion (OTEC) Biofouling and Corrosion Symposium (R.H. Gray, ed.), PNL-SA-7115, U.S. Department of Energy, Washington, D. C. 20545, pp 89-106, 1978.

7. Harrick, N.J., Internal Reflection Spectroscopy, Interscience Publishers, NY, 1967.

8. Baier, R.E., Loeb, G.I., and Wallace, G.T., Role of an Artificial Boundary in Modifying Blood Proteins, Federation Proceedings, $\underline{30}$:1523-1538, 1971.

9. Baier, R.E. and Glantz, P.O., Characterization of Oral In Vivo Films Formed on Different Types of Solid Surfaces," Acta Odontol. Scand., $\underline{36}$:289-301, 1978.

10. Baier, R.E., "Adhesion to Different Types of Biosurfaces," in Dental Plaque and Surface Interactions in the Oral Cavity (S.A. Leach, ed.), Information Retrieval Inc., Arlington, VA, pp 31-47, 1980.

11. Baier, R.E., "Substrata Influences on the Adhesion of Microorganisms and Their Resultant New Surface Properties," in Adsorption of Microorganisms to Surfaces (G. Bitton and K.C. Marshall, eds.), Wiley-Interscience Publishers, NY, pp 59-104, 1980.

12. Baier, R.E., "Occurrence, Nature and Extent of Cohesive and Adhesive Forces in Dental Integuments," Chapt. 5, Surface Chemistry and Dental Integuments (A. Lasslo and R.P. Quintana, eds.), C.C. Thomas, Publisher, Springfield, IL, pp 337-391, 1973.

13. Baier, R.E. and Loeb, G.I., "Multiple Parameters Characterizing Interfacial Films of a Protein Analogue, Polymethylglutamate," in Polymer Characterization: Interdisciplinary Approaches (C.D. Craver, ed.), Plenum Press, NY, pp 75-96, 1971.

14. Baier, R.E., "Modification of Surfaces to Reduce Fouling and/or Improve Cleaning," in *Fundamentals and Applications of Surface Phenomena Associated with Fouling and Cleaning in Food Processing* (B. Hallstrom, D.B. Lund, and Ch. Tragardh, eds.), Division of Food Engineering, Lund University, Alnarp, Sweden, pp 168-189, 1981.

15. Baier, R.E. and Meyer, A.E., "Surface Energetics and Biological Adhesion," *Proceedings, International Symposium on Physiochemical Aspects of Polymer Surfaces* (K. L. Mittal, ed.) Plenum Press, NY, 1982.

16. Baier, R.E., "Conditioning Surfaces to Suit the Biomedical Environment: Recent Progress," Journal of Biomechanical Engineering, 104:257-271, 1982.

RECEIVED April 23, 1984

# Fibrinogen-Glass Interactions: A Synopsis of Recent Research

J. L. BRASH, S. UNIYAL, B. M. C. CHAN, and A. YU

Departments of Chemical Engineering and Pathology, McMaster University, Hamilton, Ontario, Canada L8S 4L7

> A synopsis of research from the authors' laboratory over the past few years on fibrinogen-glass interactions is attempted. Relevant phenomenological data on adsorption kinetics, isotherms, desorption and exchange for the single protein system are discussed. The physical status of fibrinogen eluted from glass as evaluated by CD and polyacrylamide gel electrophoresis is also discussed and correlated with results from the phenomenological studies. It is concluded that several populations of adsorbed molecules are present on glass and that these are degraded to varying extents, probably by the action of plasmin, formed by plasminogen activation on the surface. Competitive adsorption studies with albumin and IgG in binary and ternary mixtures show a strong preferential adsorption of fibrinogen. However with plasma itself fibrinogen is not detected on glass at contact times from 2 to 180 min. It is postulated that fibrinogen is rapidly adsorbed and then desorbed, and that this transient behaviour may be mediated by the degradative action of plasmin generated at the glass surface.

The interactions of fibrinogen with glass have been a continuing topic of research in this laboratory over the past several years. In the context of studies of blood-material interactions, glass may be regarded as a model hydrophilic (water wettable) surface carrying a net negative charge at physiologic pH (SiO$^-$ groups). It has also been used extensively for handling blood and plasma in the blood coagulation laboratory and its propensity for activation of the contact phase of coagulation is well documented (1). Fibrinogen is important as the direct precursor of fibrin, the essential material of blood clot. It has also been claimed,

0097-6156/84/0256-0045$06.00/0
© 1984 American Chemical Society

notably by Vroman et al (2), that it is preferentially adsorbed from blood onto contacting foreign surfaces and several groups (3-5) have shown that adsorbed layers of fibrinogen are reactive towards platelets, causing extensive adhesion and secretion.

In our continuing studies of the glass fibrinogen system, we have investigated adsorption kinetics and isotherms from solutions of fibrinogen as a single protein in buffer (6), adsorption "equilibria" for mixtures of two or three proteins (7,8), and adsorption kinetics from plasma (9) and from buffered suspensions of red blood cells (10). We have also investigated the properties of fibrinogen that has been eluted from glass; for example, its CD spectra (11), and polyacrylamide gel electrophoresis patterns (12). In the present paper, we review the totality of these data and attempt a synthesis of our current knowledge of this system. Such a synthesis relates both to the fundamental aspects of the interaction and to its relationship to blood-material interactions, incorporating both our own work and that of others. In the context of the present Symposium this paper will serve the additional purpose of illustrating some of the principles of protein adsorption discussed in the paper of Andrade (this volume).

Kinetics and Isotherms of Adsorption - Single Protein in Buffer

In most of these studies, we have used a commercial preparation of fibrinogen from Kabi (Grade L, greater than 90% clottable), and this has normally been used after dialysis into an appropriate buffer. The experimental methods involve the use of radioiodine-labelled fibrinogen and have been described in detail elsewhere (6,9). It is merely noted here that this technique has been widely used in studies of protein adsorption (13,14), mainly to obtain an accurate measure of quantity of protein adsorbed. With this method, it is possible to determine with reasonable precision quantities of the order of a microgram and this is a typical requirement in systems where adsorption may be of the order of a fraction of a microgram per cm^2. Questions have been raised (15) as to the effects of labelling on protein behaviour. In this regard, we have established for many systems, including the glass-fibrinogen system, that iodination by the iodine monochloride method at low degrees of substitution does not influence adsorption.

In these experiments, the glass surface is in the form of Pyrex tubing, treated extensively with chromic acid followed by distilled water and then equilibrated in the buffer to be used for adsorption. The experimental design is such that measurements can be done under either static or flow conditions.

In an extensive study of the adsorption kinetics and isotherms (6), we showed (a) that the adsorption is 75% complete within 5 minutes and essentially at equilibrium in 2 hours, (b) that the kinetics between 5 and 300 minutes is not affected by shear rate up to 2100 s^{-1} in a laminar tube flow experiment, (c) that the adsorption isotherm, as shown in Figure 1, is Langmuir-like, reaching a plateau value of about 0.7 µg cm^{-2} in 0.05 M Tris, pH 7.35 at a concentration of about 0.2 mg ml^{-1} (for comparison, the plasma concentration of fibrinogen is 2-4 mg ml^{-1}), and (d) that the adsorption is irreversible in the sense that one cannot redescend the isotherm by reducing the fibrinogen concentration. This latter aspect was investigated over times of 5 h and the possibility cannot be ruled out that desorption occurs on a much longer time scale. Desorption is likely to be highly activated and therefore to be an inherently slow process. In addition binding may involve several sites on a single protein molecule as has been suggested by Morrissey and Stromberg (16) and by Jennissen (17). Desorption would then involve the simultaneous breaking of several bonds, a process of low probability.

These findings suggest that the glass-fibrinogen interaction is a strong one, since the adsorption is rapid (and not transport controlled in this experimental arrangement), the surface concentration is high (for comparison, polyethylene adsorbs about 0.2 µg cm^{-2} under similar conditions), and the adsorption is either not at all or only slowly reversible. All this notwithstanding, a determination of the free energy change based on a pseudo-equilibrium constant derived from the slope of the isotherm at zero concentration (Figure 2) (18) indicates a value of the order of -7 kcal mole^{-1}. This relatively low value may reflect non-specific binding mechanisms perhaps involving hydrophobic interactions.

However, it must be kept in mind that such a value reflects only those interactions occurring in the initial stages of adsorption at very low surface coverage. Since the glass surface is probably heterogeneous with several different types of adsorption site (see below), the initially occupied sites may not be truly representative of the surface as a whole. Also, in the intermediate and later stages of adsorption, protein-protein interactions will become important and will influence the energetics of the process.

Additional data showed (6) that in media of increased ionic strength at physiologic pH, adsorption decreases and that about 80% of the fibrinogen adsorbed from 0.05 M Tris can be eluted instantaneously with 1.0 M Tris (Figure 3). In addition, it was shown that under steady state conditions (surface concentration invariant with time), exchange occurs between adsorbed and dissolved fibrinogen but only a certain fraction of the adsorbed layer (between 30 and 70%, depending on electrolyte concentration and fibrinogen concentration) is exchangeable. Such exchange occurs with relaxation times of the order of one hour (Figure 4).

The effect of electrolyte concentration suggests binding in the adsorbed layer (protein-surface and perhaps protein-protein) is an attractive electrostatic phenomenon, since interactions of this type would be expected to diminish through the charge

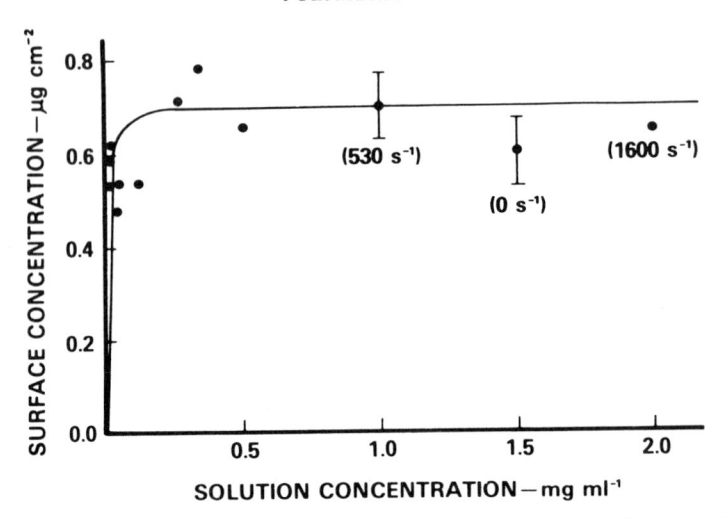

Figure 1. Adsorption isotherm of fibrinogen on glass. When not specified, data were obtained at 1060 sec^{-1}. Reproduced with permission from Ref. 6. Copyright 1981, Academic Press, Inc.

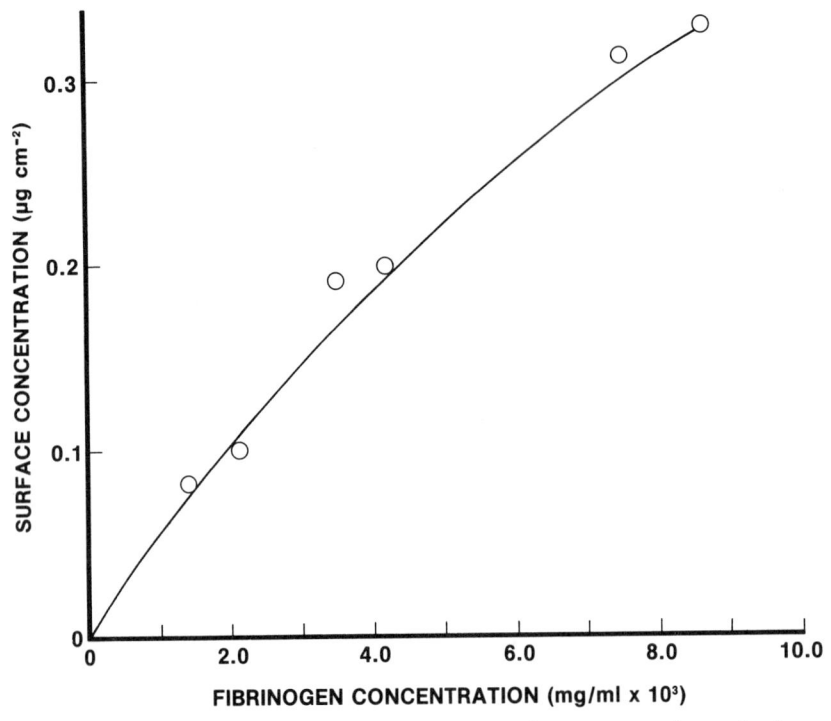

Figure 2. Adsorption isotherm of fibrinogen on glass in low concentration regime.

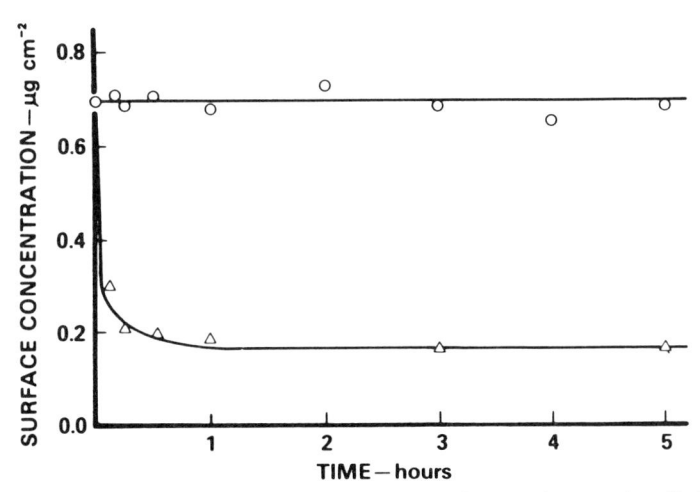

Figure 3. Desorption of fibrinogen from glass at pH 7.35 and 1060 sec^{-1}; (O) 0.05 M Tris; (Δ) 1.0 M Tris. Adsorption was from 1.0 mg ml^{-1} fibrinogen in 0.05 M Tris, pH 7.35. Reproduced with permission from Ref. 6. Copyright 1981, Academic Press, Inc.

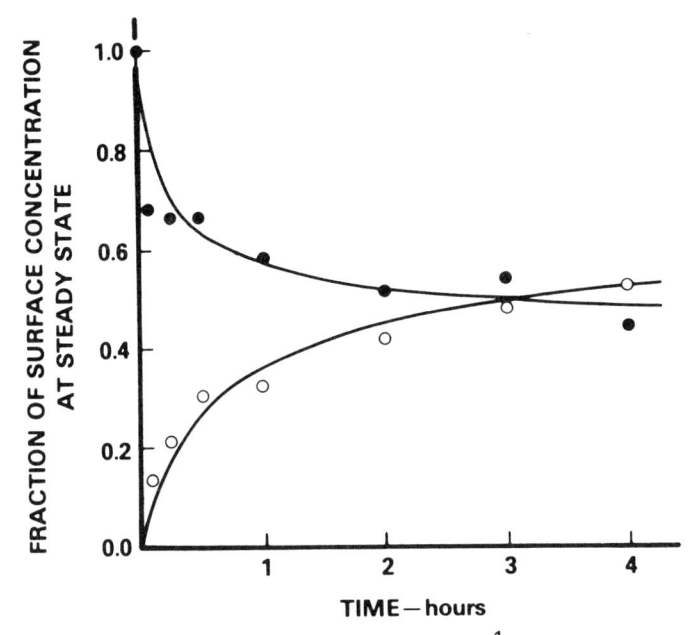

Figure 4. Turnover kinetics at 2.0 mg ml^{-1} fibrinogen, 0.05 M Tris, pH 7.35, 1060 sec^{-1}. ^{125}I-labeled fibrinogen (O); ^{131}I-labeled fibrinogen (●). Reproduced with permission from Ref. 6. Copyright 1981, Academic Press, Inc.

screening and ion exchange effects of additional ions. The occurrence of self-exchange of only a part of the layer and the partial desorption by 1 M Tris are indicative of at least two populations of adsorbed molecules, distinguished by different binding affinities. Indeed, since the fraction adsorbed or exchanged is a continuous increasing function of electrolyte concentration (6), there may well be a continuum of such populations. Such a model of the adsorption system would help to reconcile the apparent contradiction between the data suggesting strong interactions (including indications of electrostatic binding) and the relatively low free energy value, suggesting weaker interactions. As already indicated, the latter would relate to the near zero coverage regime which may be a small "non-typical" population of sites.

The fact that some self-exchange occurs may be seen as difficult to reconcile with the apparent irreversibility of the adsorption. If one takes the point of view that the adsorption is inherently reversible but that desorption occurs at a vanishingly slow rate, the question immediately arises as to why self-exchange is rapid. Since self-exchange presumably involves desorption of one molecule followed by adsorption of another, then it would be expected that desorption into buffer would occur at a similar rate to self-exchange. The major difference between the self-exchange experiment and the desorption experiment is the complete absence of solution fibrinogen in the latter. It may therefore be speculated that desorption is facilitated by the participation of protein from solution perhaps via impact collision or complex formation.

For example if adsorption involves multi-site binding then one can envisage a cooperative effect whereby a single site of an adsorbed molecule "desorbs" while a single site of a solution molecule "adsorbs" to the same surface site. Such single site exchange would represent the initiation step of whole molecule exchange. These ideas represent a simple extension of the cooperative adsorption mechanism proposed by Jennissen (17) and have been discussed in relation to self exchange by Andrade (this volume).

Our current view on reversibilty in this system, taking all the above evidence into account, is that the adsorption is inherently reversible. In addition to the self-exchange phenomenon, other evidence in support of this view is that one can "climb" the isotherm in well delineated stages: if adsorption were truly irreversible, one would expect the isotherm to rise instantly to the plateau so that in very dilute solutions (e.g., the conditions of Figure 2), complete depletion would be predicted. Since this does not occur reversibility is implied.

Structural Status of Eluted Protein

As indicated above, there appears to be a significant contribution of electrostatic interactions, whether protein-surface or protein-protein interactions, in the glass-fibrinogen system. Such strong interactions may generate interfacial forces that are sufficient to disrupt the secondary and tertiary structures of the fibrinogen molecule and therefore one might expect the occurrence of denaturation. To examine the possibility of such denaturation effects, which could have strong biological significance, we undertook studies to evaluate the structural properties of fibrinogen after elution from glass. Clearly, it would be preferable to evaluate structural alteration while the protein remains on the surface but such an approach presents formidable experimental difficulties, not the least of which is sensitivity. Therefore, we made the compromise of studying eluted protein and making the tacit assumption that the eluted protein is structurally similar to the adsorbed protein. The eluents used (high molarity buffers and surfactants) were shown not to affect the properties examined.

In one series of experiments, fibrinogen eluted from glass tubing or fritted glass filters was examined by circular dichroism (11). Controls were incorporated so that any effects of protein handling (e.g., the concentration step) could be allowed for. The eluted protein showed a loss of α-helix content of the order of 50% relative to the "native" unexposed fibrinogen, so that surface interactions appear to be capable of disrupting α-helical regions of the protein. It should be noted that we could not distinguish in these experiments between indiscriminate desorption of whole protein with an overall reduction of α-helix content and preferential desorption of portions of the molecule with inherently low α-helix content.

A second series of experiments utilizing glass bead columns was designed so that adsorbed fibrinogen could be eluted in stages (12). After adsorption from 0.05 M Tris, pH 7.4, initial fractions were eluted with 1 M Tris, which, as had been shown with labelled protein, removes 80% of the adsorbed fibrinogen. The remaining 20% (as judged by labelled protein) was eluted with 2% SDS. The fractions were examined by SDS-PAGE under reducing conditions and a typical gel is shown in Figure 5. It can be seen that the initially eluting fractions, presumably containing the fibrinogen molecules that are the least firmly bound, have undergone considerable chain degradation. It seems likely that degradation is related to contact with the glass. The extent of degradation decreases in later-eluting fractions until for the SDS-eluate, there is very little difference from "native" fibrinogen. The fact that various fractions differ in extent of degradation suggests that several surface populations are present, in agreement with conclusions based on self-exchange and differential elutability as discussed above.

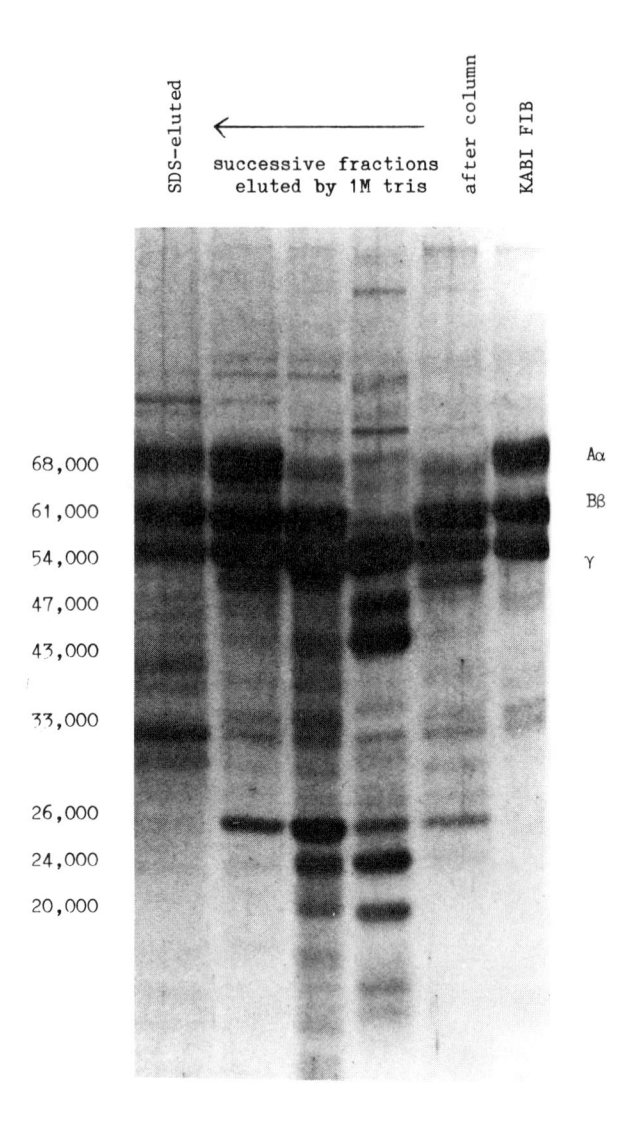

Figure 5. SDS-polyacrylamide gel electrophoresis (reducing conditions) of fibrinogen after elution from glass bead column.

All eluted samples reacted with antibody to human fibrinogen in double-diffusion experiments, indicating that the eluted material is fibrinogen-related and not an impurity concentrated on the column. Furthermore, the gel band patterns of the degraded fractions bear a strong resemblance to those of early plasmin-induced degradation products of fibrinogen (FDP). Figure 6 shows gels of FDP and column eluates for comparison. The FDP contain bands that have been attributed by Furlan and Beck (19) to fragments X and Y. Therefore, a possible explanation of our results is that traces of plasminogen present in the fibrinogen preparation are activated to plasmin by contact with glass. In this regard, we have found that fibrinogen purified on DEAE cellulose, which is reported to remove plasminogen (20), is less degraded after glass contact than is unpurified fibrinogen.

It is pertinent to mention at this point that we have recently observed similar PAGE patterns in proteins eluted from a glass bead column after contact with human plasma (21). These observations suggest rather strongly that plasminogen activation and subsequent fibrinogen degradation may be blood-material interactions of some significance that have not been recognized heretofore. This possibility will be further discussed below in relation to data on adsorption of fibrinogen from plasma.

An alternative explanation of fibrinogen degradation on glass is that adsorption renders the molecule more susceptible to hydrolytic attack (either enyzme-related or otherwise). In this regard, it is worth noting that the α-chains, which are known to be hydrophilic and to extend as random coils into the aqueous phase (22), are the most extensively degraded in all eluted fractions.

It is also instructive to compare the CD and PAGE data for the 1 M Tris eluate. It seems reasonable that chain degradation would be accompanied by changes in α-helix content, as actually observed. Unfortunately, we do not have CD data on the SDS-eluted protein which, as we have seen, is relatively undegraded. Budzynski has reported (23) that plasmin fragments D and E contain more α-helix than whole fibrinogen. On the other hand, the model recently presented by Doolittle (22) indicates that a large proportion of the α-helical content of the molecules is located in the "connector" regions between the D and E fragments, suggesting that the latter would be lower in α-helical content than the whole molecule. Regardless of which of these opposite "models" is correct, it seems likely that since the 1 M Tris eluates are much lower in α-helix content than is native fibrinogen, the degradation products eluted from glass have undergone alterations of their secondary structure due to their contact with the surface. This explanation appears more plausible than the alternative one based on preferential desorption of particular fragments that are low in α-helix and retention of others that are high.

Finally, it may be noted that the condition of the eluted protein may have a bearing on reversibility. A necessary (though not sufficient) condition of reversibility is that the protein should be capable of elution by some means (e.g., change in buffer conditions), such that it is not denatured or altered in any way (24). Otherwise, it would have to be assumed that the protein had undergone an irreversible change in the adsorbed state so that reversibility of the adsorption would be impossible. In this regard, the fact that part of the fibrinogen eluate (the later 1 M Tris and SDS eluates) is recovered in apparently unaltered form, supports the point of view that at least a part of the adsorbed layer interacts reversibly with glass.

Competitive Adsorption

In order to approach more closely to the blood system itself and to determine the influence of other proteins on fibrinogen adsorption, we undertook studies of competitive adsorption between fibrinogen and other plasma proteins. In these studies, sometimes the adsorption of only fibrinogen (labelled with ^{125}I) was followed; sometimes that of both fibrinogen and a second protein (labelled with ^{131}I) were followed.

For the binary system albumin-fibrinogen in Tris buffer (7), it was found that fibrinogen is preferentially adsorbed. In a series of mixtures of varying composition, the equilibrium ratio of surface mole fraction to solution mole fraction of fibrinogen ranged from 70 (solution mole fraction = 0.01) to 6 (solution mole fraction = 0.15). These data are illustrated in Figure 7 and emphasize the very strong fractionation effect of the glass surface with these mixtures. The results for glass can be placed in the context of other surfaces by reference to Table I.

Table I. Adsorption of Albumin and Fibrinogen to Various Surfaces. Albumin 2 mg cm^{-3} + Fibrinogen 0.05 mg cm^{-3}

Surface	Albumin Γ_A (µg cm^{-2})	Fibrinogen Γ_F (µg cm^{-2})	Mole Ratio (F:A)
Polyurethane 1200	0.330	0.083	0.051
Siliconized Glass	0.216	0.069	0.065
Polyurethane 1540	0.016	0.041	0.520
Polyurethane 600	0.013	0.055	0.859
Polystyrene	0.193	0.215	0.226
Collagen	0.097	0.213	0.446

Reproduced with permission from Ref. 25. Copyright 1979, John Wiley & Sons, Inc.

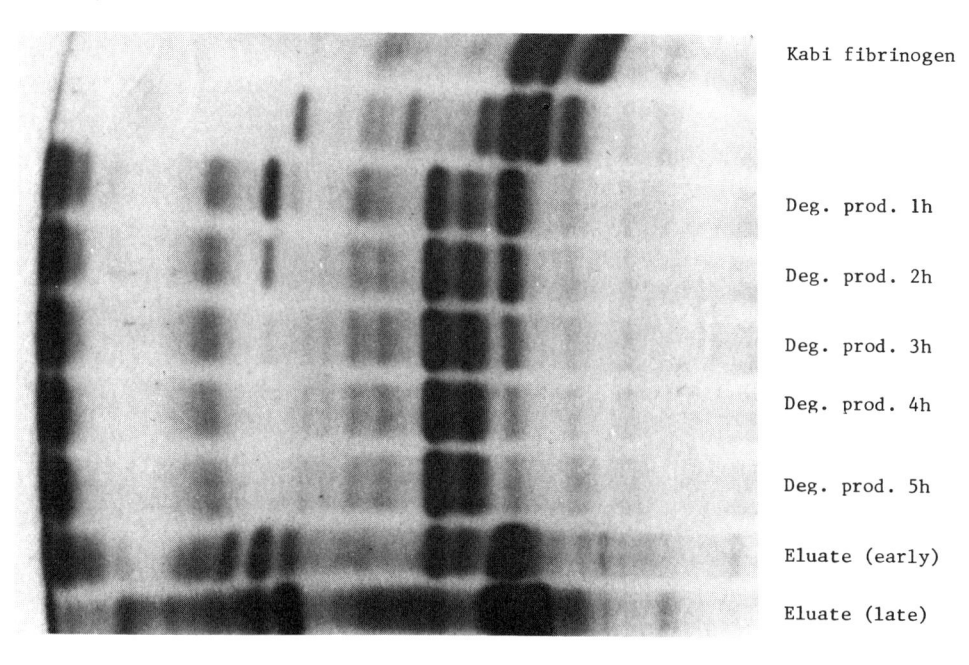

Figure 6. Comparison of plasmin degradation products with glass bead column eluate of fibrinogen.

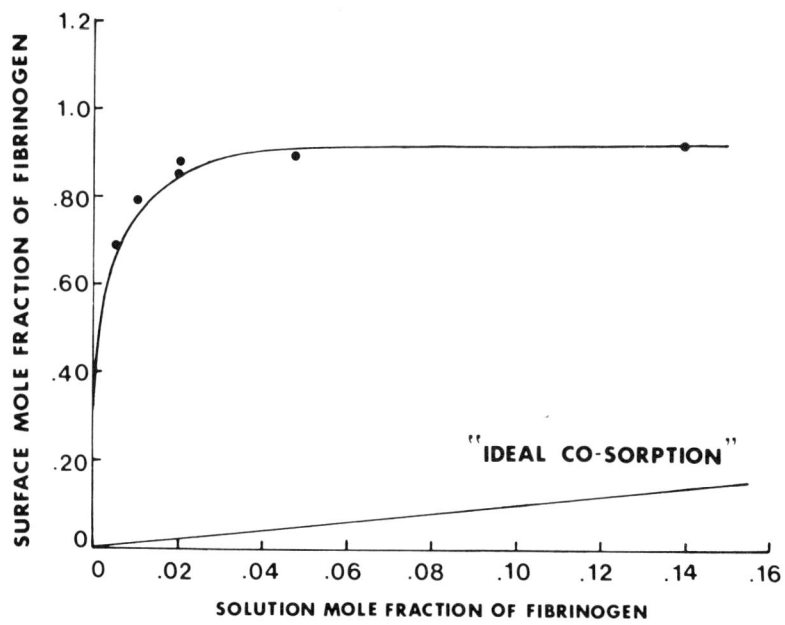

Figure 7. Adsorption on glass from various mixtures of albumin and fibrinogen. Reproduced with permission from Ref. 7. Copyright 1976, Pergamon Press, Inc.

This Table (25) gives the fibrinogen:albumin mole ratio in the layer adsorbed from solutions having a mole ratio of 0.005, close to the ratio found in normal human plasma. The surface mole ratios range from 0.05 to 0.5, reflecting a surface enrichment factor between 10 and 100. For the same solution ratio, the surface enrichment on glass is about 450.

In ternary mixtures of fibrinogen, IgG and albumin (26), the preferential adsorption of fibrinogen is again observed. These experiments were conducted using proportions of the proteins the same as are found in blood, but at varying total concentrations. For each composition, three separate kinetic experiments were conducted in which each of the three pair combinations of the proteins were labelled, and the third protein was unlabelled. Figure 8 shows typical data for the composition having the highest total concentration of protein. Over four hours, the fibrinogen adsorption increases continuously, although the rate decreases, while the IgG shows an adsorption maximum at about 5 minutes and then remains constant at a relatively low value. Albumin adsorption was effectively zero in these experiments. These data again demonstrate the overwhelming preference of glass for fibrinogen relative to the other abundant plasma proteins. Thus, it is tempting to suggest that from plasma or blood, fibrinogen would be preferentially adsorbed. This point should be kept in mind when results of adsorption from plasma are discussed below. It is also relevant to point out that the experiments with the ternary system were all conducted at total concentrations that are very dilute compared to plasma. For example, the data of Figure 8 were obtained at an albumin concentration about 3% of that in normal plasma. As will be seen below, we have recently found in plasma itself at this dilution that adsorption of fibrinogen is greatly enhanced. Thus, in retrospect, it would be desirable to conduct the ternary system experiment at or near the total concentrations in plasma before making definitive conclusions or extrapolations to plasma and blood.

Several other groups have also found preferential adsorption of fibrinogen from 2- and 3-protein mixtures (27-30). These studies have been done on a variety of surfaces with various mixture compositions and total concentrations and consistently confirm fibrinogen preferential adsorption as a general effect. Many of these measurements refer to equilibrium and involve relatively long adsorption times; information on the time dependence of relative quantities adsorbed in multi-protein systems is largely missing. One of the few such studies is that of Gendreau et al (28), using FTIR spectroscopic techniques. They found that for a 1:1, (w/w) mixture of albumin and fibrinogen, albumin predominated in the first 7 minutes and then was gradually displaced by fibrinogen. Again, these results are relevant to effects noted in adsorption from plasma, to which we now turn our attention.

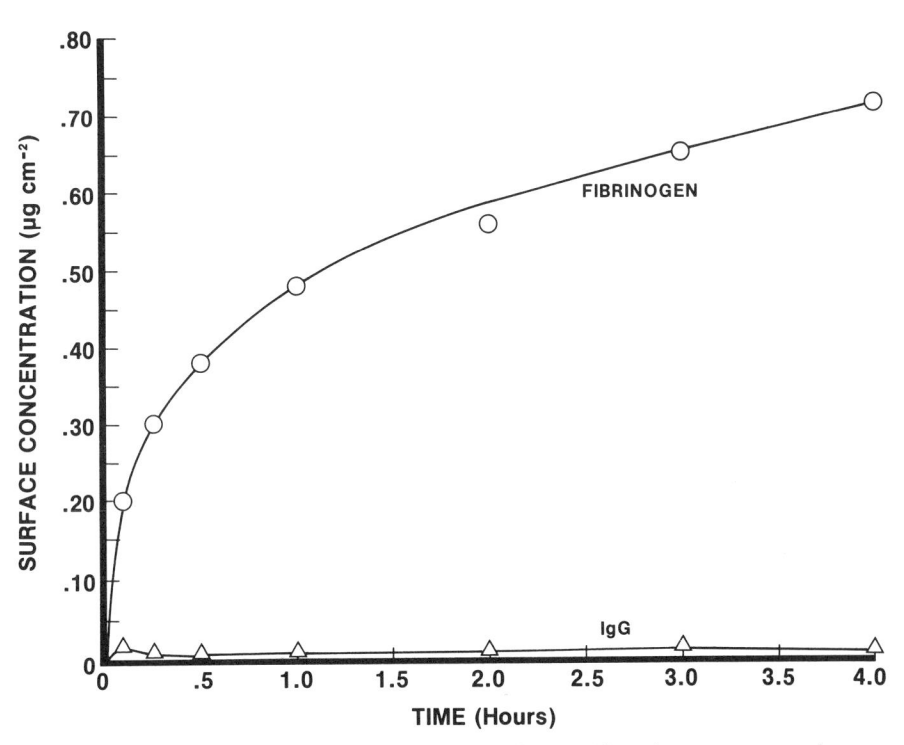

Figure 8. Adsorption on glass from the ternary system fibrinogen-albumin-IgG, concentrations 0.09, 1.20 and 0.36 mg ml^{-1} respectively. Buffer: 0.05 M Tris, pH 7.35.

Adsorption from Plasma

In these studies (9) we again utilized iodine-labelled fibrinogen added to the plasma as a tracer. The amounts of labelled fibrinogen were always less than 10% of the total amount of fibrinogen in the plasma and we have verified that the proportion of the tracer does not influence the data. Using either undiluted plasma or plasma diluted 1:4, it was concluded that essentially no fibrinogen was adsorbed to a Pyrex glass surface over a period of 4 hours. This result is surprising in view of the very substantial adsorption from single protein solutions and simple mixtures. On other surfaces (e.g., polyethylene), fibrinogen adsorbed substantially at short times (less than 2 minutes), but then desorbed almost completely over the subsequent 60 minutes. Also, fibrinogen that was pre-adsorbed from buffer was almost completely desorbed after 5 minutes of contact with plasma. These observations suggest that fibrinogen may well adsorb to glass at very short times and then be removed, possibly by exchange with other proteins or by enzymatic action.

The work of Vroman et al (31) is particularly relevant in regard to our plasma results. They have determined by various means, including ellipsometry and immunochemical techniques, that on "glass-like" surfaces, fibrinogen is adsorbed extensively during the first few seconds of contact with plasma, but is rapidly replaced by high molecular weight kininogen (HMWK), and possibly by factor XII. When the surface is exposed to very thin layers of plasma (less than 10 µm), this replacement does not occur because, it is believed, there is insufficient HMWK or factor XII (32). If this explanation is correct, then it suggests that when very dilute plasma is used, there may also not be sufficient HMWK to replace initially adsorbed fibrinogen. Recent experiments in our laboratory (33) have shown, in agreement with this point of view, that at high dilutions, there is a marked increase in fibrinogen adsorption to glass. Horbett (34) has made similar observations. Adsorption shows a maximum at a dilution of 1 to 200 and then decreases at higher dilutions. The surface concentration at maximum adsorption is about a factor of 20 higher than for 1:10 diluted plasma. It thus appears that as the absolute concentration of each species in plasma decreases, the relative amounts of these proteins in the surface layer changes even though the relative amounts in the plasma remain the same. Such an effect could result from different shaped isotherms for the different proteins in plasma. For example, the absolute concentrations at which the isotherm plateaux are reached is almost certainly different for the various proteins so that increases in adsorption of some proteins and decreases in others will occur as a function of plasma dilution. If this explanation is correct, it would be of interest to determine which of the multitude of proteins in plasma decreases as fibrinogen increases in the adsorbed layer. These proteins would presumably be important components of the adsorbed layer in normal undiluted plasma.

Additional information on plasma-fibrinogen-glass interactions has been obtained by examining the eluates from glass bead columns after plasma contact (21). Essentially, undiluted ACD-human plasma is loaded on the column and allowed to equilibrate. After washing out residual plasma, the columns are sequentially eluted with 1 M Tris and 2% SDS. SDS-PAGE of eluted proteins shows complex banding patterns. This work is as yet at a very preliminary stage and no definite conclusions have been reached as to the identity of the eluted proteins. The M.W. patterns are, however, very strongly suggestive of plasmin-induced degradation products and the 1 M Tris eluates give precipitation lines in Ouchterlony double immunodiffusion experiments with anti-human fibrinogen. In agreement with the earlier results for "pure" fibrinogen, these data again suggest the possible activation of plasminogen on glass surface and its subsequent attack of adsorbed fibrinogen. Further experiments are underway to check this possibility.

For the moment some speculation may be permissible regarding a possible connection between this degradation effect and the time transients in fibrinogen adsorption from plasma observed by Vroman et al and implied in data from this laboratory. As already indicated, Vroman et al attribute the time-transient effect to replacement by HMWK, but it could equally well be that it is due in the first instance to the action of surface-generated plasmin in facilitating desorption via degradation and that this is potentiated by HMWK. The dilution effect would then be seen as the result of having insufficient plasminogen and HMWK to cause degradation and desorption. These hypotheses could be tested by working with plasmas deficient in plasminogen and/or HMWK. Addition of inhibitors of the plasminogen-plasmin system to normal plasma would also provide useful information to help resolve these questions.

Acknowledgments

The financial support of our research by the Medical Research Council of Canada and the Ontario Heart Foundation over the past several years is gratefully acknowledged.

Literature Cited

1. Cochrane, C.G.; Griffin, J.H. Amer. J. Med. 1979, 67, 657-64.
2. Vroman, L.; Adams, A.L.; Klings, M. Fed. Proc. 1971, 30, 1494.
3. Packham, M.A.; Evans, G.; Glynn, M.F.; Mustard, J.F. J. Lab. Clin. Med., 1969, 73, 686-697.

4. Lyman, D.J.; Klein, K.G.; Brash, J.L.; Fritzinger, B.K.; Andrade, J.D.; Bonomo, F. Thromb. Diath. Haemorrhag. 1971, Suppl. 42, 109.
5. Whicher, S.J.; Brash, J.L. J. Biomed. Mater. Res. 1978, 12, 181-201.
6. Chan, B.M.C.; Brash, J.L. J. Colloid Interface Sci., 1981, 82, 217-25.
7. Brash, J.L.; Davidson, V.J. Thromb. Res. 1976, 9, 249-59.
8. Yu, A.; Brash, J.L., unpublished observations.
9. Uniyal, S.; Brash, J.L. Thromb. Haemostas. 1982, 47, 285-90.
10. Uniyal, S.; Brash, J.L.; Degterev, I.A., in "Biomaterials: Interfacial Phenomena and Applications"; Cooper, S.L.,; Peppas, N.A., Eds.; ADVANCES IN CHEMISTRY SERIES No. 199, American Chemical Society; Washington D.C., 1982; p. 277.
11. Chan, B.M.C.; Brash, J.L. J. Colloid Interface Sci., 1981, 84, 263-5.
12. Brash, J.L.; Chan, B.M.C. Trans. Soc. Biomaterials 1982, 5, 85.
13. Horbett, T.A. J. Biomed. Mater. Res., 1981, 15, 673-95.
14. Young, B.R.; Lambrecht, L.K.; Cooper, S.L.; Mosher, D.F. In "Biomaterials: Interfacial Phenomena and Applications"; Cooper, S.L.; Peppas, N.A., Eds.; ADVANCES IN CHEMISTRY SERIES No. 199, American Chemical Society; Washington, D.C., 1982; p. 317.
15. Crandall, R.E.; Janatova, J.; Andrade, J.D. Preparative Biochem. 1981, 11, 111-138.
16. Morrissey, B.W.; Stromberg, R.R. J. Colloid Interface Sci. 1974, 46, 152-64.
17. Jennissen, H.P. Biochemistry 1976, 15, 5683-92.
18. Schmitt, A.; Varoqui, R.; Uniyal, S.; Brash, J.L.; Pusineri, C. J. Colloid Interface Sci. 1983, 92, 25-34.
19. Furlan, M.; Beck, E.A. Biochem. Biophys. Acta. 1972, 263, 631-44.
20. Lawrie, J.S.; Ross, J.; Kemp, G.D. Biochem. Soc. Trans. 1979, 7, 693-4.
21. Brash, J.L.; Szota, P., unpublished observations.
22. Doolittle, R.F. Scientific American 1981, 245, 126-35.
23. Budzynski, A.Z. Biochem. Biophys. Acta 1971, 229, 663-71.
24. One of us (J.L.B.) is indebted to M. Jozefowicz on this point.
25. Brash, J.L.; Uniyal, S., J. Polymer Sci. 1979, C66, 377-89.
26. Yu, A.; Brash, J.L., unpublished observations.
27. Lee, R.G.; Adamson, C.; Kim, S.W. Thromb. Res. 1974, 4, 485-90.
28. Gendreau, R.M., Leininger, R.I.; Winters, S.; Jakobsen, R.J. In "Biomaterials: Interfacial Phenomena and Applications"; Cooper, S.L.; Peppas, N.A., Eds.; ADVANCES IN CHEMISTRY SERIES No. 199, American Chemical Society; Washington, D.C., 1982; p. 371.
29. Lok, B.K.; Cheng, Y-L.; Robertson, C.R. J. Colloid Interface Sci. 1983, 91, 104-16.

30. Horbett, T.A.; Hoffman, A.S. In "Applied Chemistry at Protein Interfaces"; Baier, R.E., Ed.; ADVANCES IN CHEMISTRY SERIES No. 145; American Chemical Society; Washington, D.C., 1975; p. 230.
31. Vroman, L.; Adams, A.L.; Fischer, G.C.; Munoz, P.C. Blood 1980, 55, 156-59.
32. Vroman, L.; Adams, A.L.; Fischer, G.C.; Munoz, P.C.; Stanford, M. In "Biomaterials: Interfacial Phenomena and Applications"; Cooper, S.L.; Peppas, N.A., Eds.; ADVANCES IN CHEMISTRY SERIES No. 199, American Chemical Society; Washington, D.C., 1982; p. 265.
33. Brash, J.L.; ten Hove, P. Thromb. Haemostas., to be published.
34. Horbett, T.A. Thromb. Haemostas., to be published.

RECEIVED March 19, 1984

6

Silicones in Artificial Organs

E. E. FRISCH

Dow Corning Corporation, Midland, MI 48640

Starting with the silicone elastomer hydrocephalus shunt in 1955, silicone elastomer has become widely used as a soft, flexible, elastomeric material of construction for artificial organs and implants for the human body. When prepared with controls to assure its duplication and freedom from contamination, specific formulations have excellent biocompatibility, biodurability, and a long history of clinical safety. Properties can be varied to meet the needs in many different implant applications. Silicone elastomer can be fabricated in a wide variety of forms and shapes by most all of the techniques used to fabricate thermosetting elastomers. Radiopacity can be increased by fillers such as barium sulfate or powdered metals. It can be sterilized by ethylene oxide, steam autoclave, dry heat, or radiation. Shelf-life at ambient conditions is indefinite. When implanted the host reaction is typically limited to encapsulation of the implant in fibrous tissue. Silicone elastomer implants have become used in essentially all surgical specialties including neurosurgery, ophthalmology, plastic surgery, urology, orthopaedic surgery, obstetrics and gynecology, otolaryngology, cardiovascular surgery, and others. Significant advances have been made in silicone elastomer technology in recent years. A medical grade high performance silicone elastomer with excellent resistance to tear propagation and fatigue flexing has been developed and qualified for use in the implants used in bone and joint reconstruction. Properties, biocompatibility, biodurability and medical applications for silicone elastomers will be discussed.

0097-6156/84/0256-0063$09.75/0
© 1984 American Chemical Society

Silicone is the common name for polydiorganosiloxanes. The term allegedly originated because it was thought silicon-containing materials first prepared by Kipping(1) at about the turn of the century might be silicon-containing analogues of ketones.

$$C(CH_3)_2=O \qquad -[Si(CH_3)_2O-]_x$$
Acetone　　　　　　　　Polydimethylsiloxane

Modern processes for syntheses of silicones were developed from research conducted in the 1930's. Silicones were first manufactured in quantity during World War II for the U. S. government to improve the performance of U. S. aircraft. After World War II and prior to distribution for other than aircraft use, animal studies were undertaken to evaluate biological characteristics. The findings indicated that non-volatile methyl- and mixed methyl- phenylpolysiloxanes as a class were very low in toxicity. Also, finished silicone resins were physiologically inert and presented no health hazards. Publication (2-3) of the study stimulated interest in using silicones for artificial organs because of the need for implantable, biocompatible, soft, flexible, elastomeric materials. This paper will review the chemistry, the physical and biological characteristics, and applications of silicones in artificial organs.

CHEMISTRY

The synthesis of silicone starts with naturally occurring silicon dioxide (quartz, sand, or quartzite rock). Silicon dioxide is reacted with carbon at high temperature to yield elemental silicon.

$$SiO_2 + C \xrightarrow{\Delta} Si + CO_2$$

The hard, crystalline, brittle elemental silicon is pulverized and reacted directly with methyl chloride at elevated temperature.

$$Si + CH_3Cl \xrightarrow{\Delta} SiCl_4 + CH_3SiCl_3 + (CH_3)_2SiCl_2 + (CH_3)_3SiCl + (CH_3)_4Si$$

A mixture of methyl- and chlorine-containing silanes ranging from tetrachlorosilane to tetramethylsilane is obtained. Conditions are generally adjusted to produce a maximum amount of dimethyldichlorosilane, the monomer for polydimethylsiloxanes. The liquified silanes are separated by fractional distillation.

Polydimethylsiloxane is prepared by condensation copolymerization of dimethyldichlorosilane with water.

$$x\,(CH_3)_2SiCl_2 + x\,H_2O \longrightarrow -[Si(CH_3)_2O-]_x + 2x\,HCl$$

The prepolymer thus obtained is further polymerized to yield specific silicone polymers which can vary in molecular weight (average and distribution), presence or absence and content of fillers or other additives, type of organic ligands attached to silicon, the possible presence of reactive radicals such as vinyl ligands on silicon for use in cross-linking, and in other ways. About 60,000 silicon-containing compounds are known. However, only a few have been found to be useful and have thus become commercially available. Silicones used in artificial organs and implants have primarily been the polydimethylsiloxanes.

Hydrocephalus Shunt

Holter's successful development of a silicone elastomer hydrocephalus shunt (4) (Figures 1-2) in 1955 heralded the era of implants. No effective treatment for hydrocephalus was known at the time. Thus, by 1957, only two years after the shunt was first used, and continuing today, essentially every hydrocephalic child born in the developed countries of the world has received a silicone elastomer hydrocephalus shunt implant. Hydrocephalus occurs in approximately one out of every 400 to 600 children born alive. The hydrocephalus shunt is one of the oldest, and also one of the most widely used of all silicone elastomer implants. Some individuals have now had shunt implants for more than 25 years. The excellent biocompatibility of implant grades of silicone elastomer is evidenced by the essential absence of adverse biological response in this long term, large volume use.

Medical Grade Silicone Elastomers

Medical grade silicone elastomers became available in the early 1960's. "Medical grade" refers to silicone elastomers specifically formulated, manufactured and qualified for implant uses. The formulations contain no materials with potential for biodegradation or adverse biocompatibility. Manufacturing and processing are done under carefully controlled, clean conditions to assure batch-to-batch duplication, and freedom from adulteration, contamination, and cross contamination. Batch-to-batch tests include assessment of chemical, physical, and biological properties. The materials must elicit no cytotoxic reaction by direct contact tissue-cell culture testing (5,6). Qualification of a controlled formulation for implant use typically requires 2-year minimum biocompatibility (host and tissue reaction) (7) and 2-year biodurability (implant reaction) studies.

High-consistency thermosetting medical grade silicone elastomer compounds are prepared from high molecular weight polydiorganosiloxanes compounded with high-surface fumed silica (approximately 400 m^2/g). Silica is the only material known that adequately reinforces silicone elastomer.

Vulcanization requires cross-linking polymer chains. In one

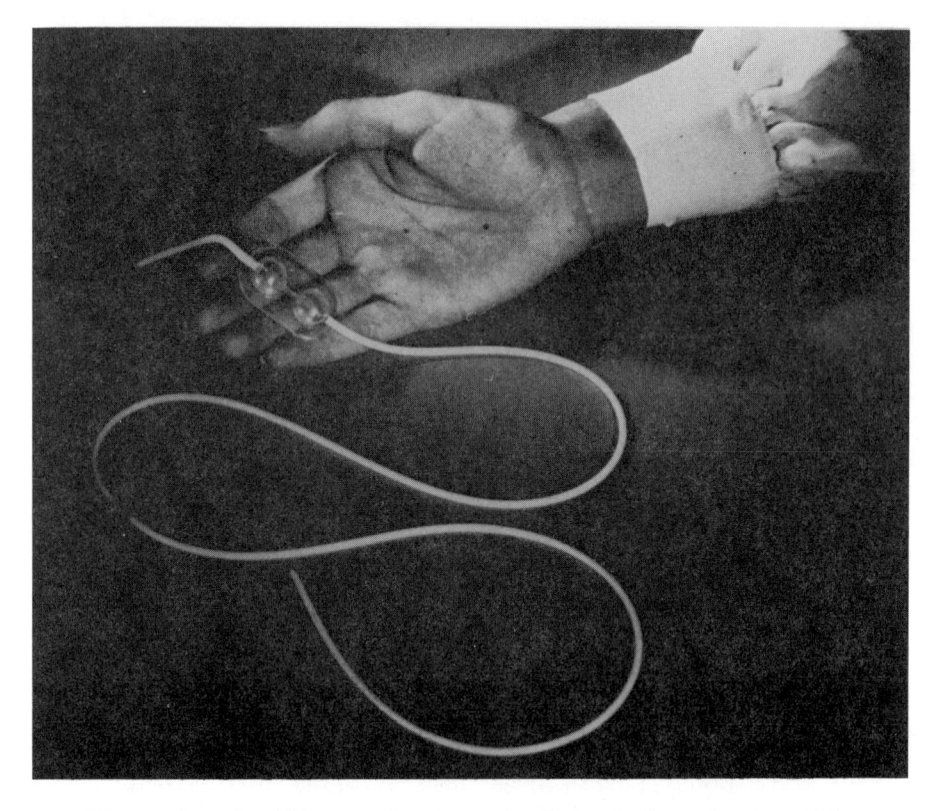

Figure 1. A silicone elastomer hydrocephalus shunt. This type of shunt is used to drain cerebrospinal fluid from the ventricle of the brain to either the vascular system or to the peritoneal cavity. The first hydrocephalus shunt was developed by Holter in 1955. The shunt in this illustration contains a dual flushing chamber to assure continual function of the shunt, and is designed to drain cerebral spinal fluid from the ventricle of the brain to the peritoneal cavity.

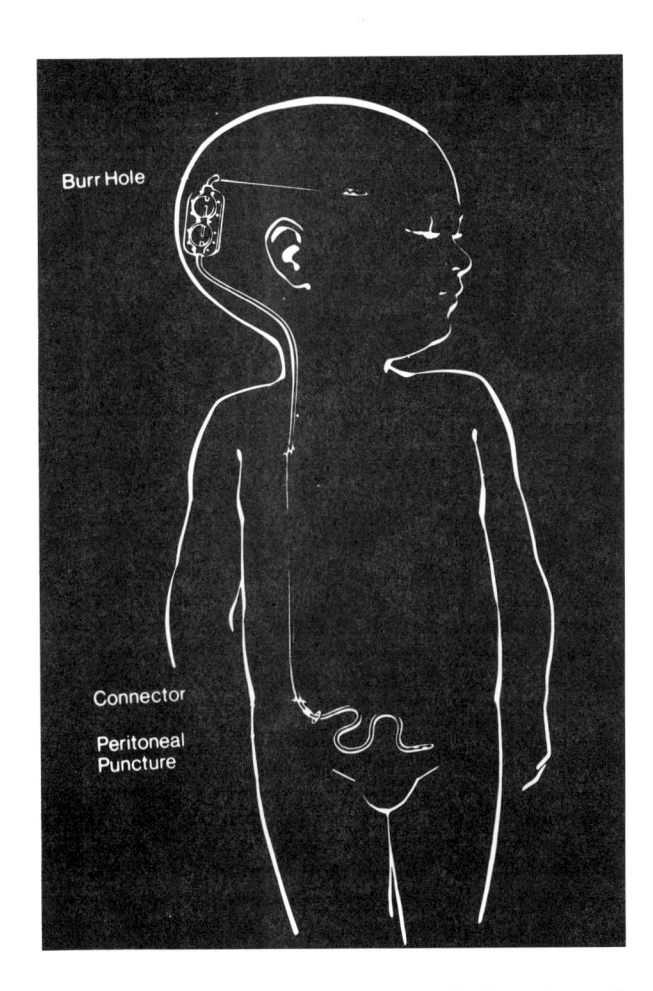

Figure 2. Positioning of the hydrocephalus shunt in a child's body. The entire shunt is implanted subdermally. The tip of the shunt is inserted into the ventricle of the brain through a hole made in the skull, while the drainage catheter is placed in the peritoneal cavity through a small incision in the peritoneal lining. An extra length of the peritoneal catheter is generally left so that the child may grow without dislodging the catheter from the peritoneal cavity.

type of cross-linking, silicon-hydrogen ligands, contained as small amounts of methylhydrogensiloxy copolymer in one formulation, react with silicon-vinyl ligands, contained as methylvinylsiloxy copolymer in small amounts in a second formulation. When the two formulations are intimately blended and heated in the presence of a catalyst, cross-linking occurs. Typical catalysts include trace quantities of rare metals, such as platinum. The cross-links are dimethylene radicals covalently bonded between silicon atoms in separate polymer chains.

Cross-linking essentially forms a chemically bonded network matrix of one giant molecule. Organic peroxides are also used as vulcanization catalysts.

Biocompatibility of Medical Grade Silicone Elastomers

When once formulated or processed silicone elastomer cannot be adequately characterized by short term studies to guarantee that historic animal and clinical data are relevant to assure reasonable safety for implant use. Unlike some substances where analysis and acute evaluations can provide thorough characterization chemical, physical, and acute biocompatibility tests, used alone or in combination, are not adequate. Formulation errors or contamination, which could adversely affect chronic biocompatibility characteristics, may inadvertently occur and not be detected by short-term testing. When used in implants reasonable assurance of duplication must include characterization of all basic ingredients, control of the manufacturing processes, and stringent quality assurance. All formulation, compounding, and processing of elastomers must be done in facilities which comply with Good Manufacturing Practice Regulations as a minimum. Silicone elastomer prepared under less stringent conditions, such as those typically used to produce elastomer for industrial use cannot be adequately upgraded by after-the-fact short-term testing to assure that chronic biocompatibility characteristics have been duplicated.

The chronic biocompatibility and biodurability of medical grade silicone elastomers have been evaluated. In one study specimens of medical grade silicone elastomer were implanted in purebred beagle dogs for 3 years. Tissue reactions typically included an initial inflammatory reaction associated with the introduction of a foreign material. The reaction appeared to be self-limiting and further diminished with time, leaving a definable fibrous capsule around the implant as the terminal observation. The most noticeable fibrous-tissue responses were caused by the intramuscular implants, with less intense reactions respectively in subcutaneous and intraperitoneal sites. The results of testing done on clinical laboratory specimens collected during the terminal weeks of the 3-year implantation study for evaluation of clinical chemistry indicated that all values were within normal limits for the species, with no abnormalities detected. The gross and microscopic findings in tissues taken at autopsy revealed no pattern of polymer-induced systemic toxicity.

In a study with albino rats specimens of test materials were implanted in a group of 100 rats, consisting of 50 males and 50 females. Similar groups, serving as controls, received implants of USP polyethylene and sham surgery only. The study was continued for the lifetime of the animals, or 2 years, whichever occurred first. Mortality data revealed no significant differences between test, treated control, or control groups with respect to the frequency or number of deaths. There were no untoward behavioral reactions in any of the animals. Histopathological evaluations revealed that tissue changes found in treated rats were similar to those in control rats. The type and incidence of neoplasms observed were considered normal for the laboratory rats of the age and strain involved in this study. None of the neoplasms observed were attributable to the experimental procedures.

Biodurability was assessed by a 2-year subcutaneous implantation study in dogs ($\underline{8}$). The study found no significant changes in physical properties of silicone elastomer as a result of 2 years of subcutaneous implantation.

Thus, medical grade silicone elastomers are biodurable, noncytotoxic, nonallergenic, nonpyrogenic, noncarcinogenic, nontoxic, and nonirritating. When implanted, the reaction is limited to a mild foreign-body reaction and encapsulation of the implant in fibrous tissue as a normal physiological response.

Physical Properties of Medical Grade Silicone Elastomers

The earlier medical grade silicone elastomers varied primarily in durometer (Shore A, ASTM 2240) from a low of about 30 to a high of about 70 (soft, medium and firm grades). Durometer was varied primarily by increasing or decreasing filler content. Other physical properties varied essentially as expected. However, as the elastomers became used in applications where physical property requirements were more demanding, such as in the implants used in bone and joint reconstruction ($\underline{9}$), the performance of conventional medical grade elastomers was no longer adequate.

Technology for substantially increasing tear propagation strength and resistance to flaw propagation during fatigue flexing was developed in the early 1970's allowing the development of medical grade high performance silicone elastomer. Crack growth resistance evaluations were done by ASTM D813. In this test a DeMattia specimen is fatigue flexed sharply at the precut flexion groove through a 180° bend. The growth of an initial through-and-through 2 mm (0.080 inch) cut is monitored as the specimen is flexed 10^6 cycles, or until the cut grows to 12.7 mm (0.5) whichever occurs first. With conventional medium hardness medical grade silicone elastomer the length of the cut typically equalled or exceeded 12.7 mm at 7333 cycles, with an extrapolated cut growth rate equal to approximately 1459 mm (57.3 inches) per 10^6 cycles. By comparison, with medical grade high performance silicone elastomer the typical cut growth rate was 2.5 mm (0.1 inch) at 10^6 cycles (reduced by a factor of approximately 570).

Listed in Table I are typical physical properties of medical grade high performance and conventional silicone elastomer.

Flex-life studies were conducted on preflawed finger joints. Before testing, a 1.57 mm (0.0652 inch) through-and-through cut was made in the center of the implant hinge. The plane of the cut was perpendicular to the long axis of the implant. Implants fabricated from conventional medical grade silicone elastomer typically separated completely by 90,000 flexes. By comparison, implants fabricated from high performance medical grade silicone elastomer routinely flexed 9 million times with an increase in flaw size but without separation. Thus, in vitro flex-life in flawed finger joints was increased more than 100 times.

After qualification by acute and chronic biocompatibility and biodurability evaluations, clinical studies were conducted to confirm that the implants were highly durable. Medical grade high performance silicone elastomer has now become used in various biomedical applications including construction of flexible bone and joint implants as designed by Swanson (9) (Figures 3-8).

Applications for Medical Grade Silicone Elastomers

Artificial organs and implants fabricated from silicone elastomer have allowed or improved treatment of a variety of human health conditions where no equally effective treatment is otherwise available.

Plastic & Reconstructive Surgery
The implants used in plastic and reconstructive surgery serve as space-occupying tissue and organ substitutes in applications that result in contour or cosmetic changes. The hardness can be varied within limits to simulate the texture of tissues replaced. Implants used in reconstruction of the nose and chin (11,12) (Figures 9-11) are usually relatively firm to simulate bone. The ear implant (13) (Figures 12-14) is flexible to simulate cartilage. The implants used for breast reconstruction (14) (Figures 15-20) typically contain a solid, thin silicone elastomer envelope (fabricated from dispersion) and filled with a soft, cross-linked silicone gel to simulate the texture of breast tissue. Custom implants from either solid silicone elastomer, or of the silicone gel type may also be prepared to meet one-of-a-kind contour needs with specific patients.

Ophthalmology
Silicone elastomer in both solid and sponge form is used as a

Table I. Typical Physical Properties of Medical Grade High Performance and Conventional Silicone Elastomer

Property	ASTM	High Performance	Medium Hardness
Tensile	D412	8.274 MPa (1200 psi)	6.895 MPa (1000psi)
Elongation	D412	700%	500%
Modulus at 100%	D412	2.413 MPa (350 psi)	2.068 MPa (300psi)
Tear, Die C	D624	52.54 k N/m (300 ppi)	Varies widely
Tear, Die B	D624	52.54 k N/m (300 ppi)	13.13 k N/m(75ppi)
Crack growth, 10^6 cycles	D813	2.5 mm (0.1 inch)	1459 (57.3 inch), Extrapolated
Durometer, Shore A	D2240	52	50
Specific gravity	D924	1.15	1.14

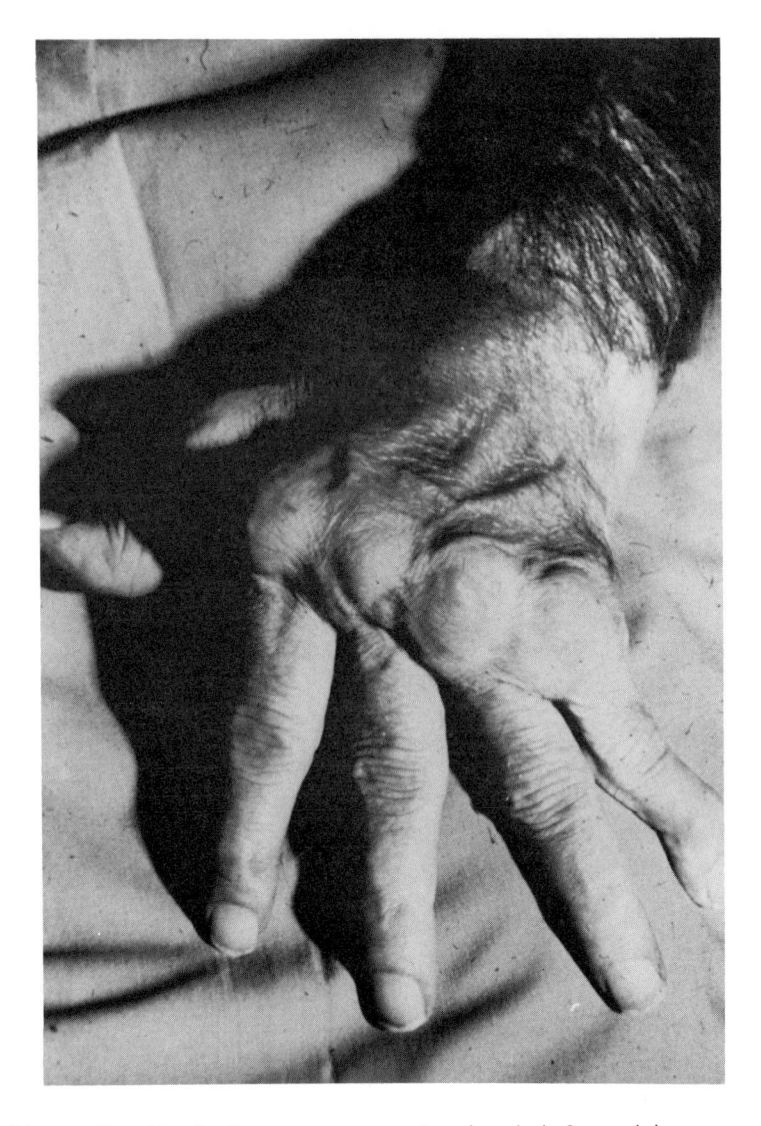

Figure 3. Typical appearance of a hand deformed by rheumatoid arthritis and a candidate for reconstruction by implant resection arthroplasty. Ulnar deviation and subluxation in the metatarsophalangeal joints, and deformity of the thumb are evident.

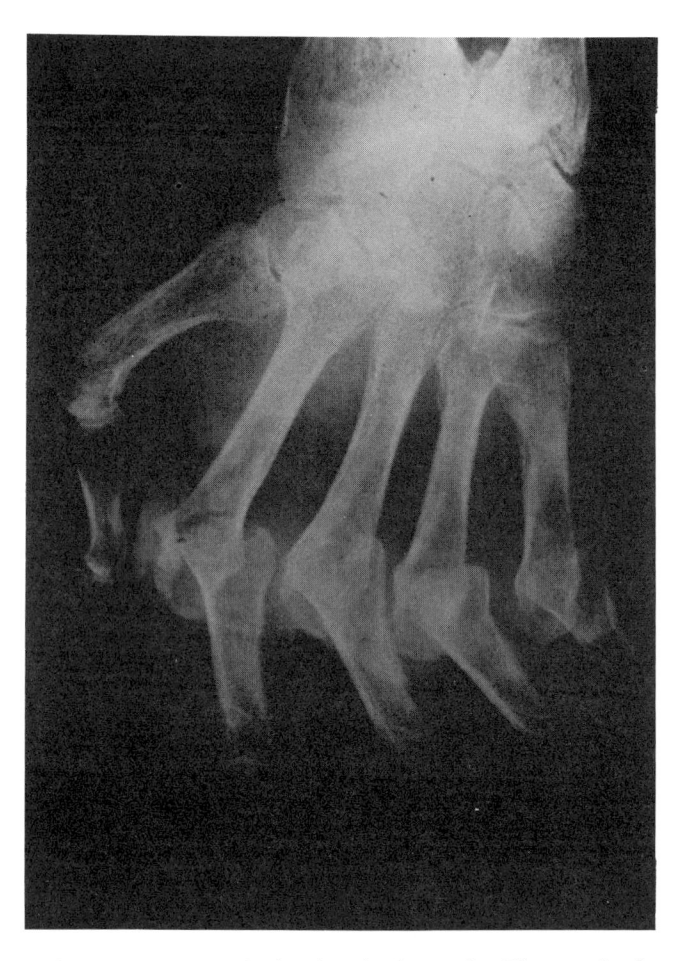

Figure 4. An x-ray of the hand shown in Figure 3 clearly illustrates the extent of the deformities.

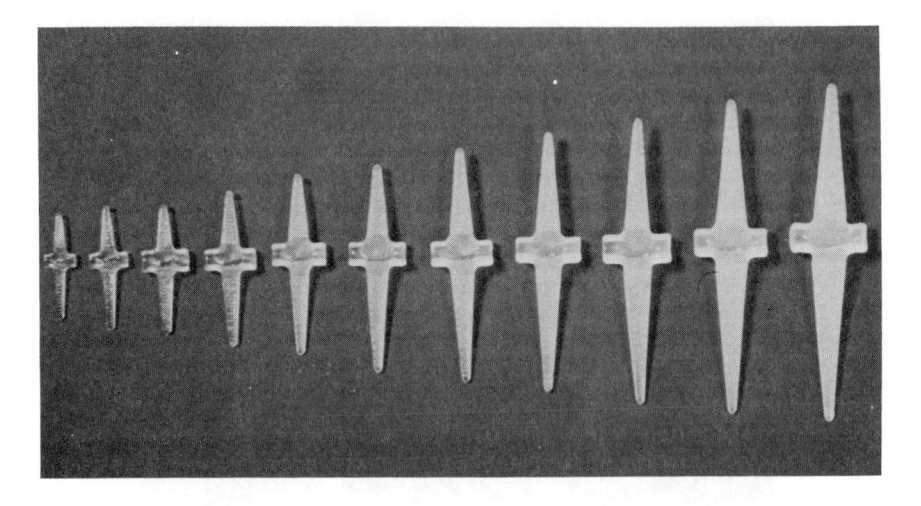

Figure 5. Flexible hinge finger joint implants designed by Alfred B. Swanson, M.D. for use in reconstruction of diseased or destroyed finger joints. The high flexural durability of these implants is derived from the design of the load-distributing hinge and the flexural fatigue resistance of medical grade high performance silicone elastomer.

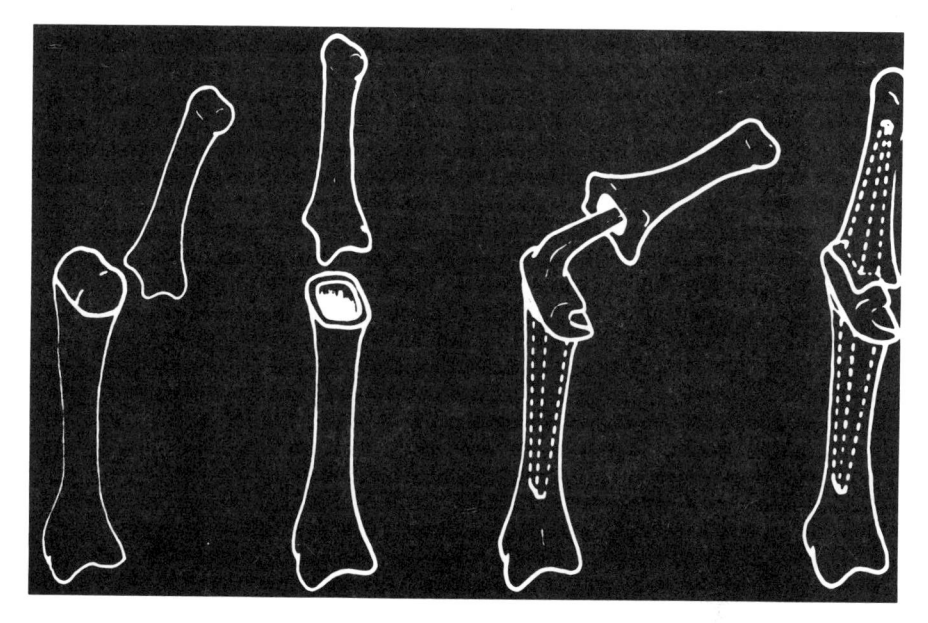

Figure 6. Surgical placement of the flexible hinge finger joint implant. The metacarpal head is removed to create an appropriate joint space and the intramedullary canals are then prepared to accept the implant stems. When the implant is placed in position the stems fit securely in the intramedullary canals with the flexible hinge permitting 90° active motion. Joint space is maintained by transfer of the compressive forces of joint motion across the implant to cortical bone. Careful attention to reconstructions of tendons, ligaments, and joint capsules and postoperative therapy are very important in this procedure.

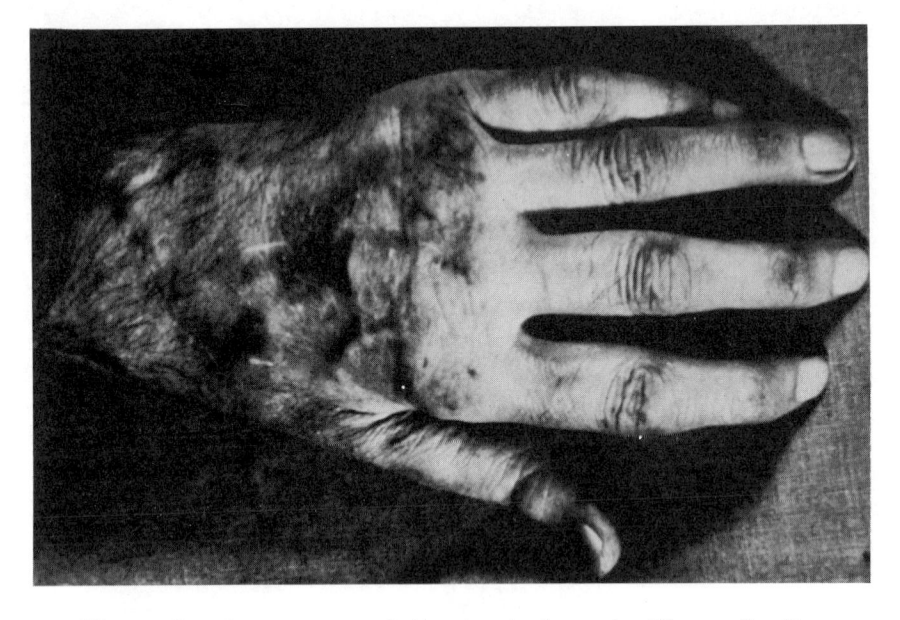

Figure 7. Appearance of the hand shown in Figure 3 after reconstruction. The hand now has essentially a normal appearance, is pain-free, mobile, and functional.

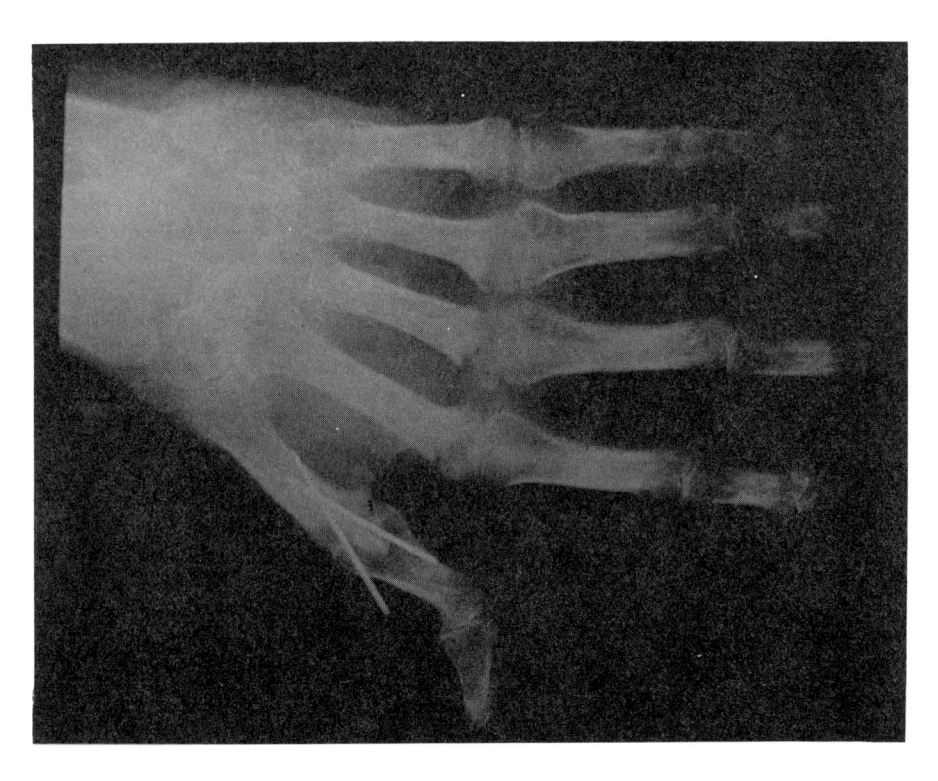

Figure 8. An x-ray of the hand shown in Figure 7 with implants in all of the metatarsophalangeal joints. Correction of deformity in the thumb included fusion of the interphalangeal joint to provide a strong pinch strength. Postoperatively, the patient returned to gainful employment. The illustrations shown in Figures 3-8 are courtesy Alfred B. Swanson, M.D.

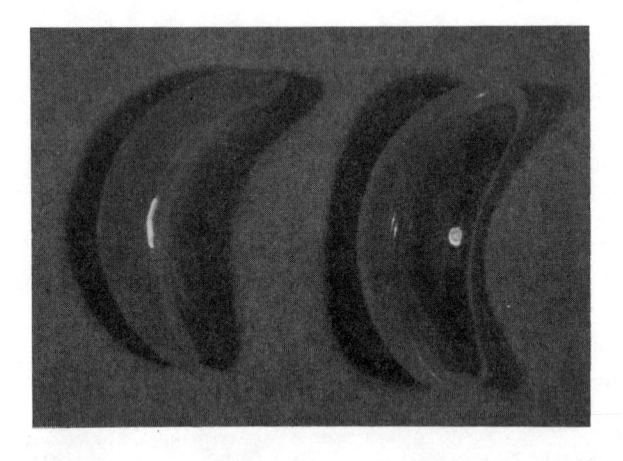

Figure 9. Chin implants molded from medical grade silicone elastomer to increase the projection of the mandible.

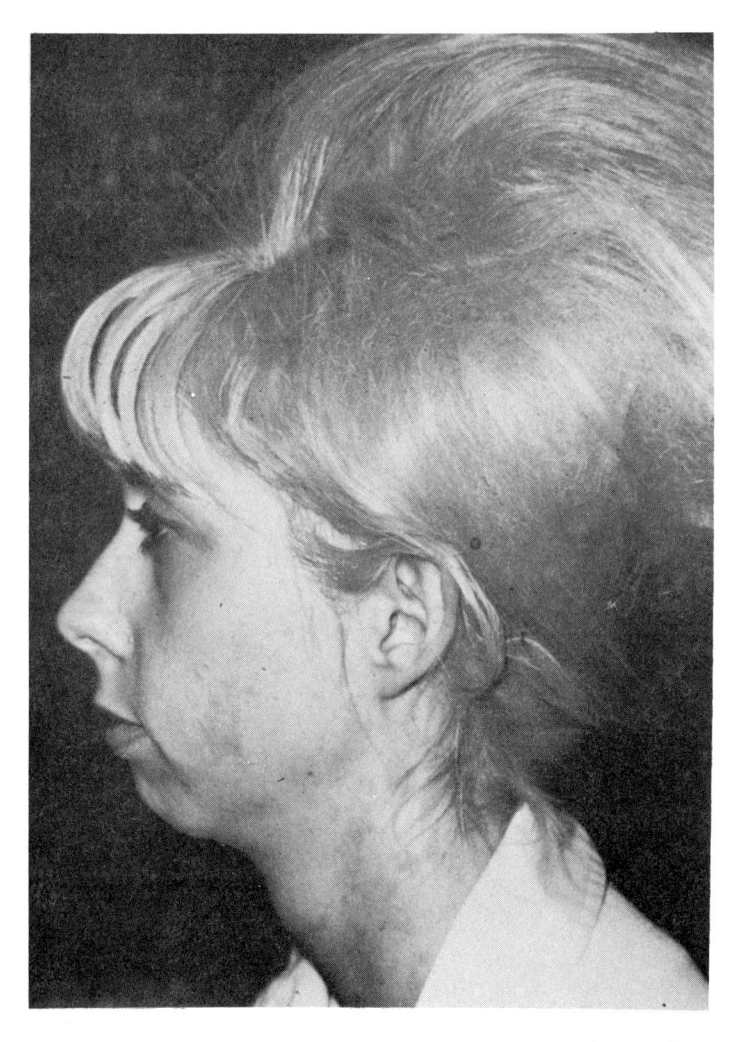

Figure 10. Preoperative appearance of a patient who believed her quality of life would be improved by a chin augmentation.

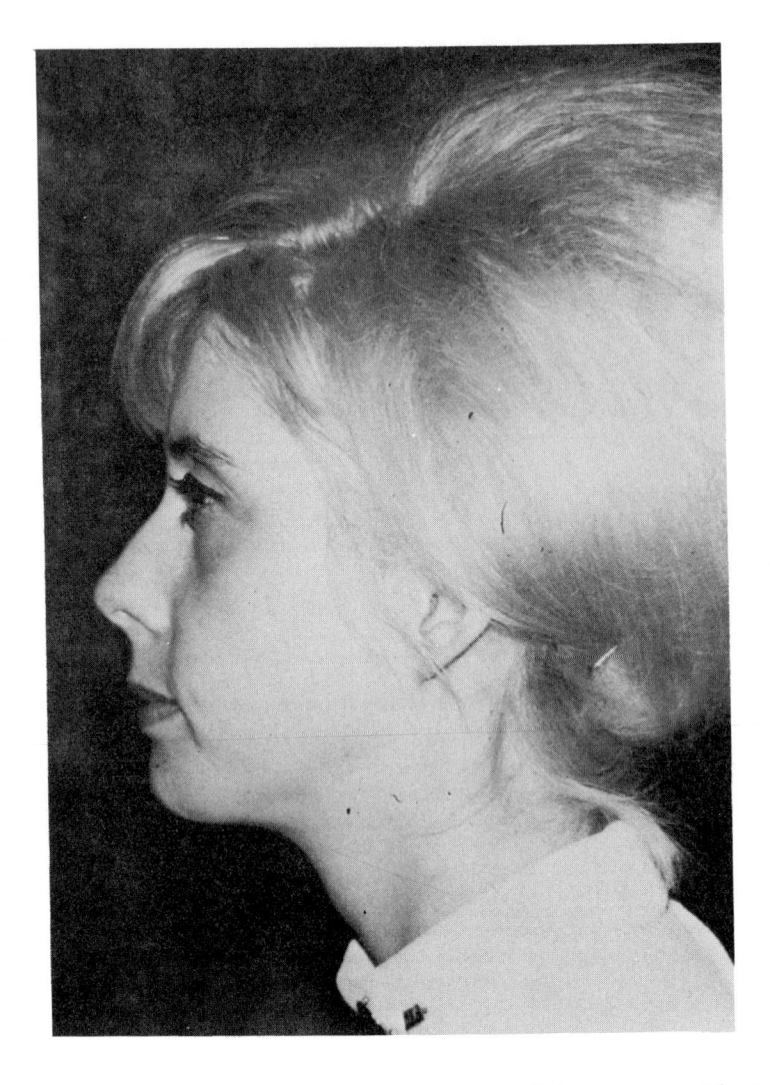

Figure 11. Postoperative appearance of the same patient shown in Figure 10.

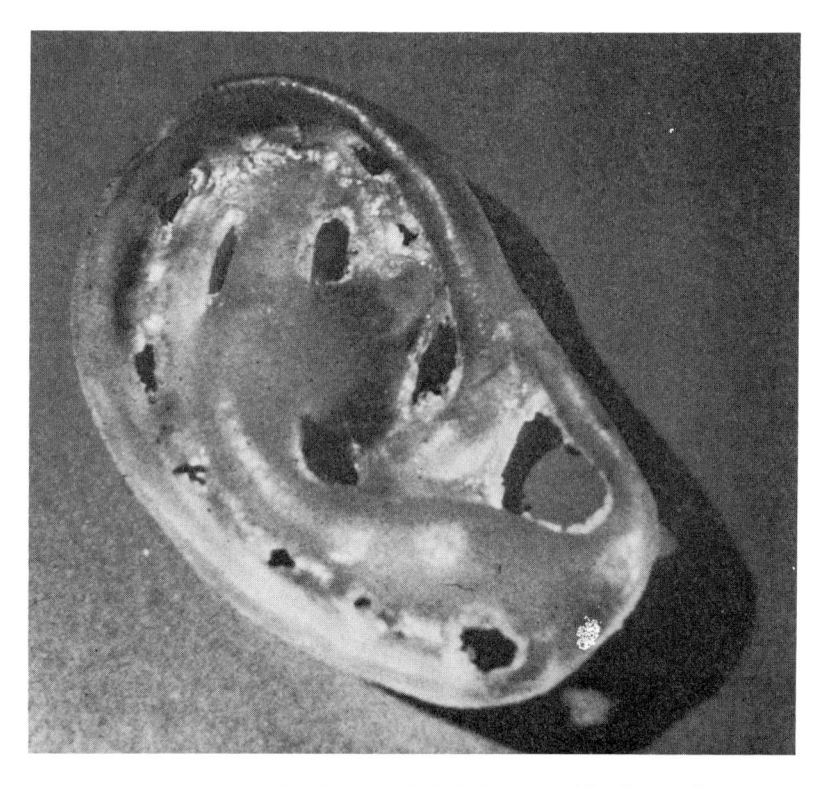

Figure 12. An ear implant molded from medical grade silicone elastomer and used as artificial cartilage in ear reconstruction.

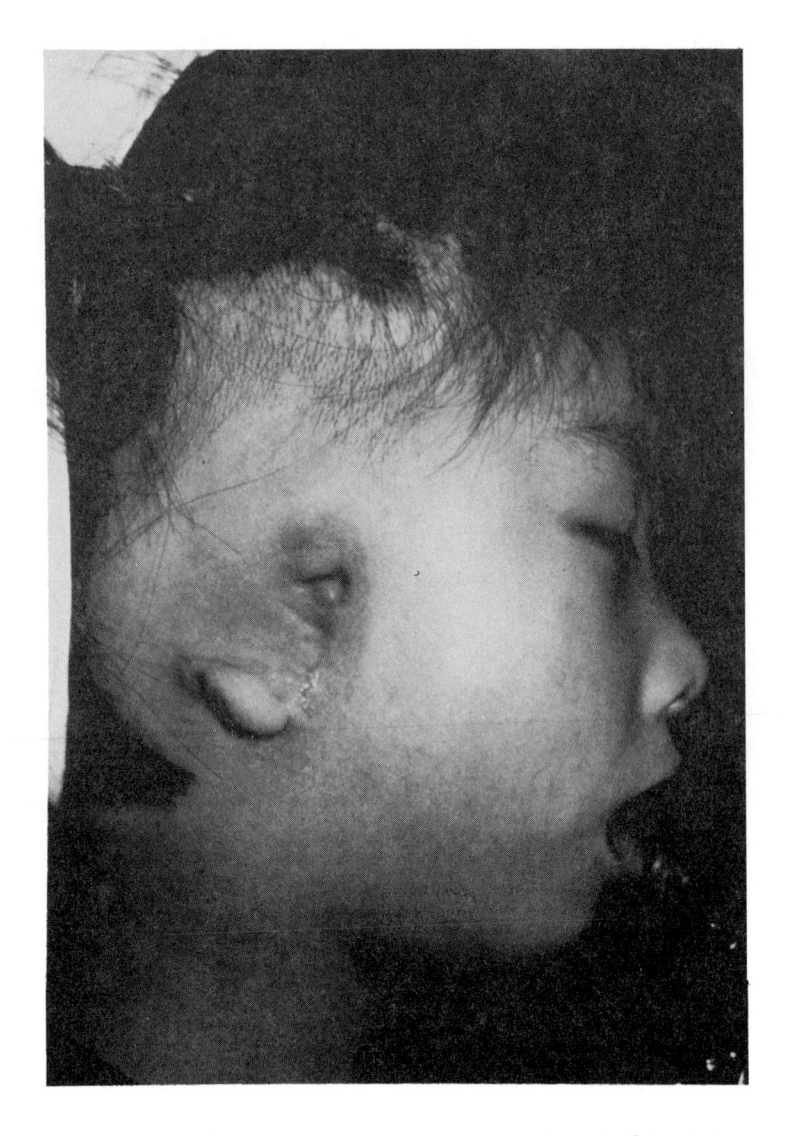

Figure 13. Preoperative appearance of a child with a missing ear.

6. FRISCH *Silicones in Artificial Organs*

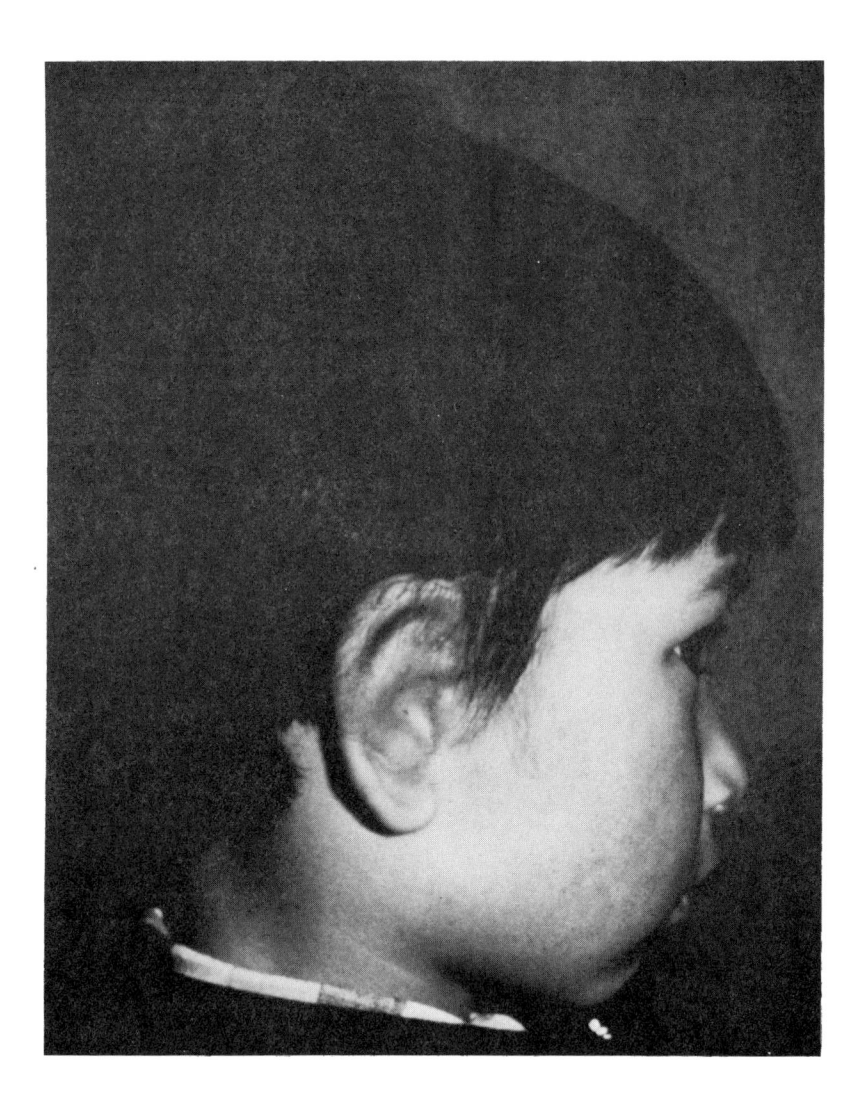

Figure 14. Postoperative appearance of the same child shown in Figure 13 following ear reconstruction with the silicone elastomer implant. His own subcutaneous tissue and skin were shaped around the silicone framework during the process of ear reconstruction.

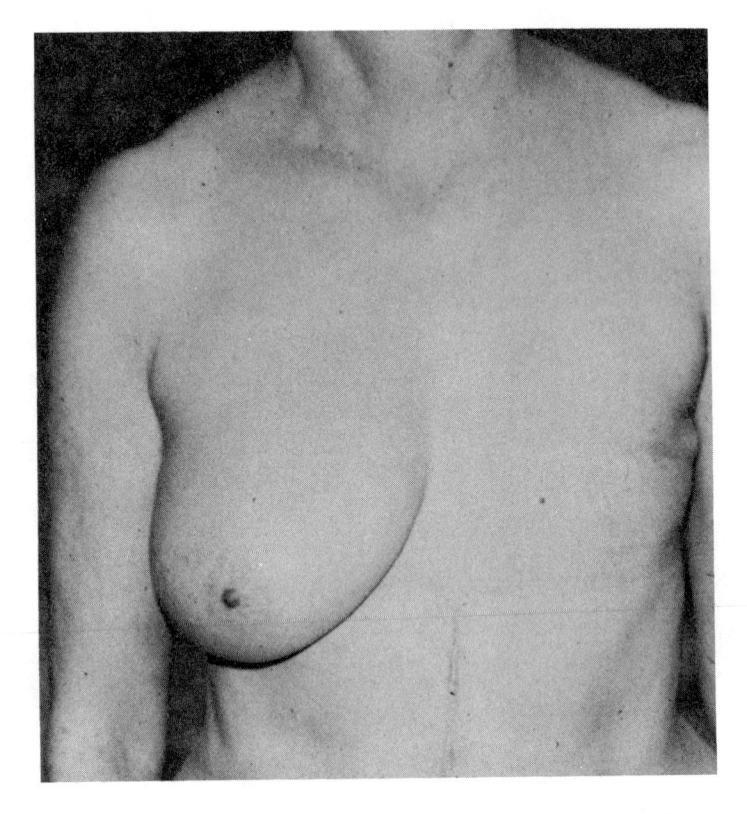

Figure 15. Preoperative appearance of a patient who has undergone a unilateral mastectomy for carcinoma of the breast.

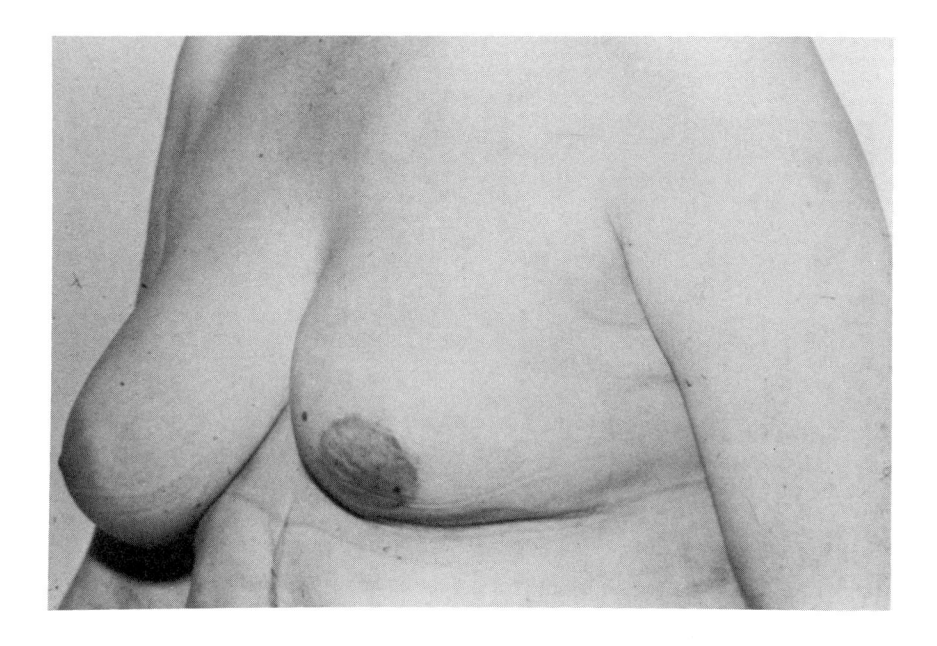

Figure 16. Appearance of the patient shown in Figure 16 following reconstruction of a breast shape with a silicone-gel type mammary implant. The nipple may be reconstructed by either a split thickness skin graft from the remaining nipple, or the color can be established by tattooing.

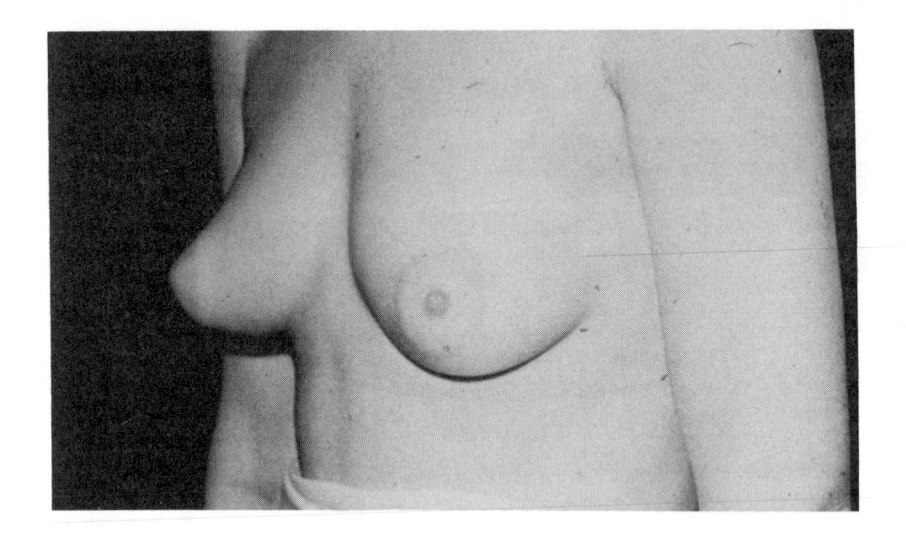

Figure 17. Preoperative appearance of a patient with chronic cystic mastitis and a family history of breast cancer, making her a high risk patient and a candidate for prophylactic subcutaneous mastectomy to substantively reduce the potential of developing carcinoma of the breast.

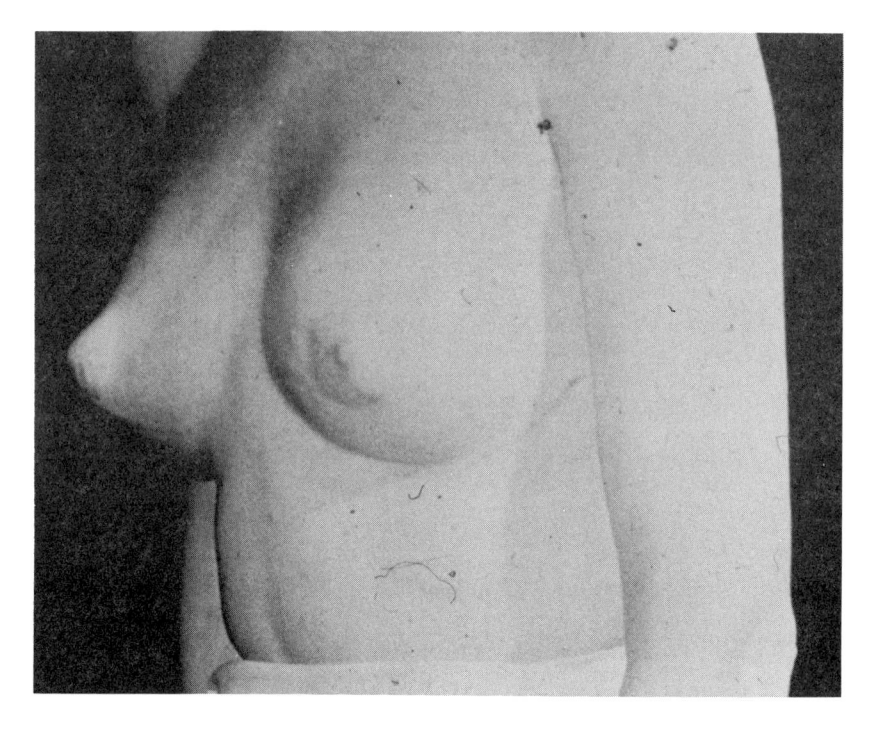

Figure 18. Postoperative appearance of the patient shown in Figure 17 following simple subcutaneous mastectomy with replacement of breast tissue by silicone-gel mammary implants.

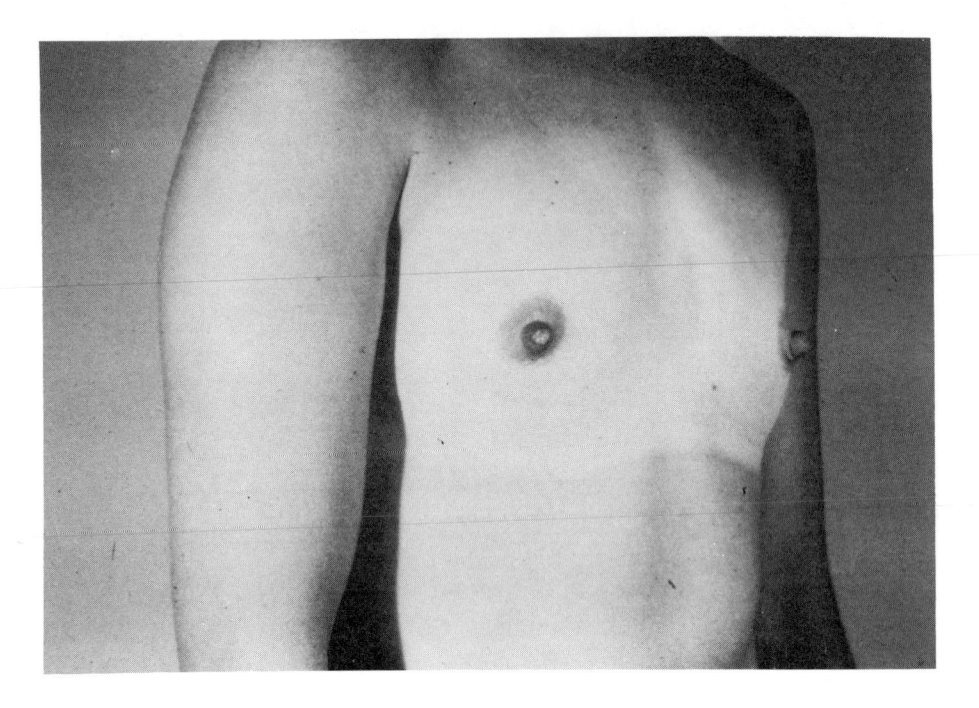

Figure 19. Preoperative appearance of an adult female patient who has not developed normal female breast contour.

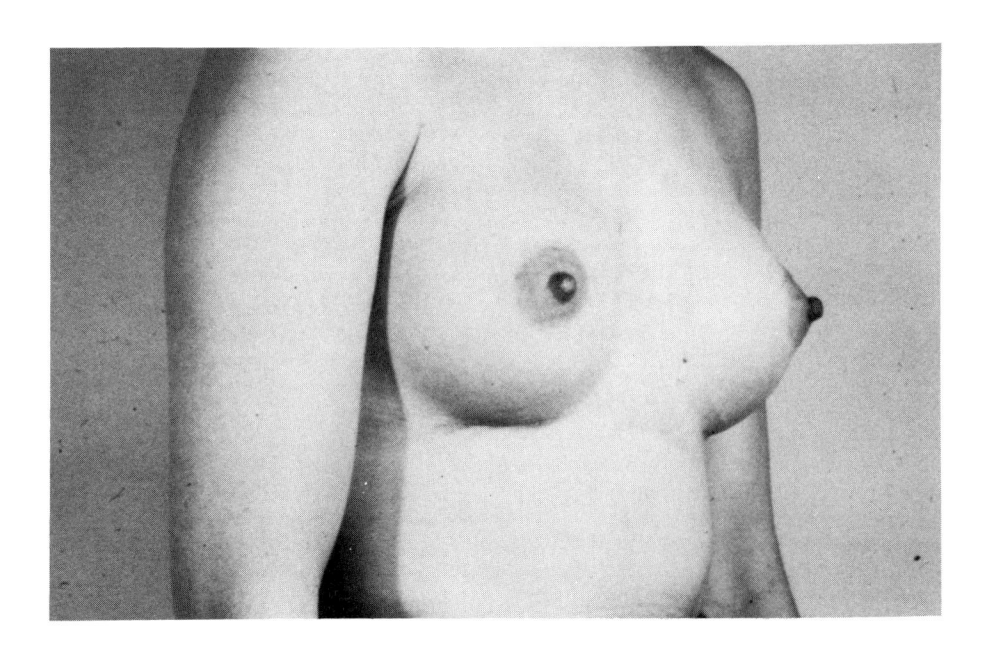

Figure 20. Postoperative appearance of the patient shown in Figure 19 following breast reconstruction with silicone-gel mammary implants.

space-occupying implant to buckle the sclera for treatment of a detached retina (10) (Figures 21-22). Silicone implants are used in repairing fracture of the floor of the orbit. Space-occupying implants are also used following enucleation to fill or adjust the void left by removal of the eye, allowing a prosthetic eye to be worn. Silicone elastomer tubes are often used to restore patency to blocked or destroyed lacrimal ducts.

Orthopaedic Surgery

A variety of flexible silicone elastomer implants have been developed (9) for reconstruction of diseased or destroyed small joints of the body. A total of 14 different implants have been developed, each in a range of sizes, for reconstruction of fingers, thumbs, wrists, elbows, and feet. The devices include a passive tendon implant used in 2-stage procedures for reconstruction of tendons. Finger, wrist, and toe joint implants are available with flexible hinges. All bone and joint implants have intramedullary stems which aid in positioning the implants and help maintain the implant spacer in correct anatomical position. The implants are fabricated from medical grade high performance silicone elastomer to provide maximum durability.

Cardiovascular Surgery

One of the earliest uses of medical grade silicone elastomer in cardiovascular surgery was for the ball in the ball-and-cage heart valve (Figure 23). In the early 1960's some of these valves failed because of swelling of the silicone elastomer balls due to absorption of lipid-type substances from the blood. This resulted in either loss of ball motion because of a tight fit within the cage, or fragmentation of the balls. However; the difficulties were traced to improper processing of the silicone elastomer, and when these processing difficulties were corrected these types of problems with silicone elastomer heart valve balls have not recurred.

Other cardiovascular uses have included coatings on pacemakers and pacemaker lead-wires for purposes of insulation and for achieving biocompatibility. Medical grade silicone elastomer has been widely used as a material of construction in experimental artificial hearts and heart assist devices. Silicone tubing is often preferred for use in roller-type blood pumps during cardiopulmonary bypass. Medical grade silicone elastomer contains no leachable or organic plasticizers and thus contributes minimal contamination in blood contact applications.

Medical Applications for Silicone Fluid

The biomedical characteristics of medical grade silicone fluid (liquid polydimethylsiloxanes) have become widely misunderstood. This is primarily because of the publicity given in both the lay and professional press to complications arising from "silicone

6. FRISCH *Silicones in Artificial Organs*

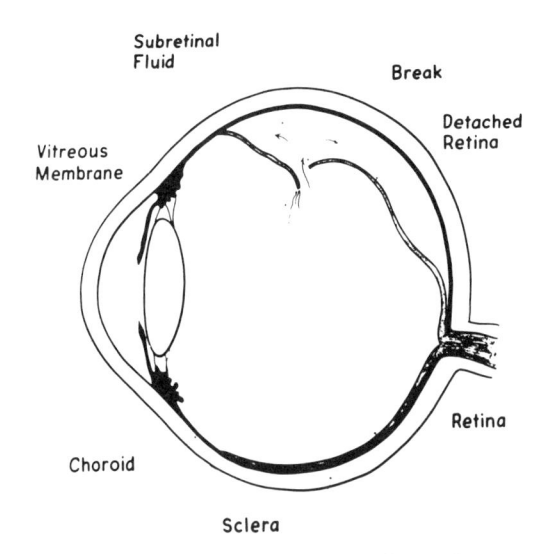

Figure 21. Drawing of a cross-section of an eye with detached retina which typically results in loss of vision and retinal deterioration.

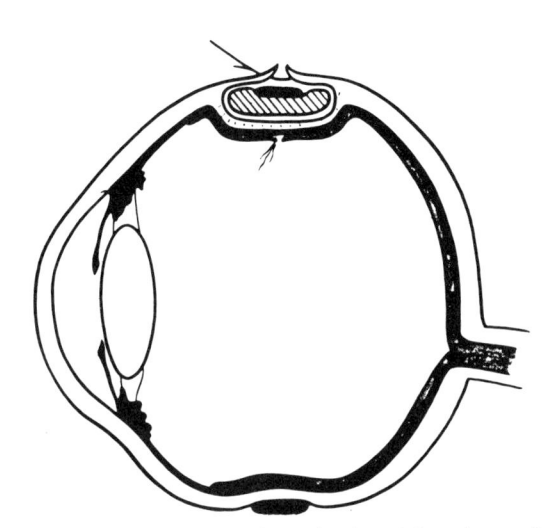

Figure 22. Correction of detached retina by scleral buckling. A silicone elastomer band completely encircles the eye to increase intraoccular pressure. An extra pad of medical grade silicone is often used beneath the band at the point of detachment in order to buckle the sclera inward and place it in contact with the retina. Reattachment may be encouraged by laser beam or diathermy stimulation.

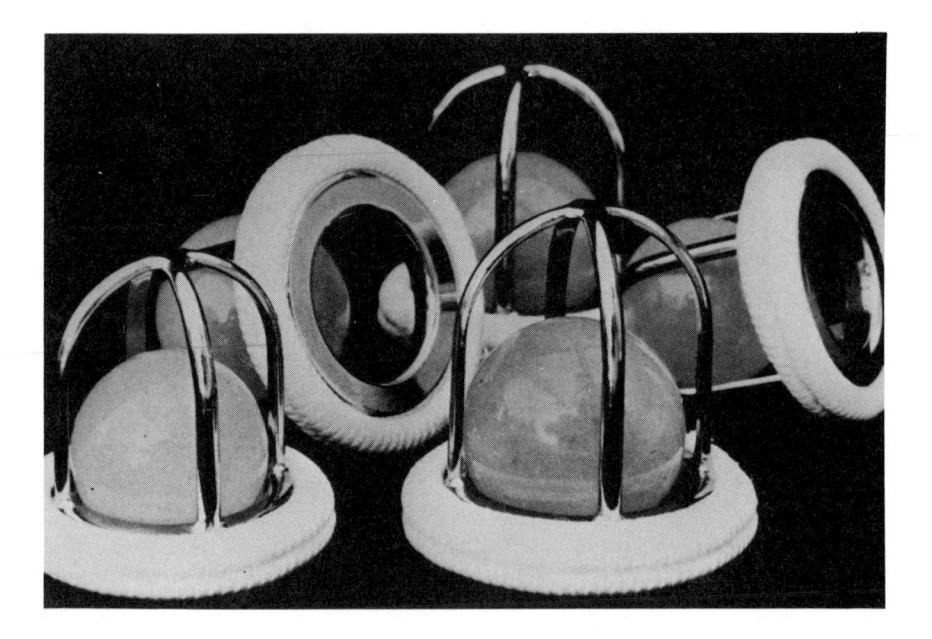

Figure 23. Ball-and-cage heart valves constructed with silicone elastomer balls. Compared to metal or rigid plastic balls, silicone elastomer balls create no noise as the heart beats. Problems from swelling and fragmentation of the balls which occurred in a few patients in the mid-1960's were traceable to the processing techniques used in fabricating balls, and when once corrected the problems have not recurred. Silicone balls continue to be used in heart valves.

fluid" injections. Injection is a serious misuse since no manufacturer recommends injection as a use for silicone fluid, and no silicone fluid has been approved via the FDA premarket approval application process for use as an injectable. Furthermore, many of the complications resulted from the injection of non-silicone or industrial silicone materials and were done under uncontrolled, scientifically unsound conditions. Those making the injections typically represented to their patients that the material being injected was "medical grade silicone fluid" without regard for its actual composition.

Essentially all injection misuses involved subdermal injection for purposes of soft tissue augmentation. Many of the complications reported were associated with injections into the female breast. By comparison, in controlled clinical investigations (where injections into the female breast were specifically excluded), done in keeping with regulatory procedures, clinical evidence has suggested that medical grade silicone fluid may, in selected cases properly done by a trained physician, be reasonably safe and effective for soft tissue augmentation by injection. However; a demonstration of safety and efficacy as required for premarket approval by FDA has not been accomplished. Accordingly, no silicone fluid should be administered to humans by injection for any purpose unless done as part of a controlled clinical investigation and done in keeping with all of the regulatory provisions.

In the interim there are other important health care applications for silicone fluids. Many of these involve its use as a lubricant. The availability of silicone fluid as a lubricant for use on disposable hypodermic needles (Figure 24) contributed to the development of the disposable hypodermic needle. Essentially all disposable hypodermic needles are lubricated with silicone fluid to permit easy insertion and removal, and to minimize pain. Prior to the use of silicone fluid lubricants disposable needles tended to be very painful and sometimes broke or bent upon insertion.

Silicone fluid is also used to lubricate disposable hypodermic syringes (Figure 25). Without a suitable lubricant it is unlikely that the disposable hypodermic syringe would have become available. Silicone fluid lubricants allow the rubber plunger tip to slide easily down the molded plastic barrel while it continues to provide a tight seal to prevent leakage of the material being injected or inflow of air upon aspiration. Syringes thus lubricated may be stored for long periods of time without change in the lubricity properties or the force required for plunger movement, very important considerations in the control over the speed and volume with which injections are given.

With each injection a small amount of silicone is deposited in the patient's tissue from the needle, and also from the syringe. However; studies (15) suggest that in these small

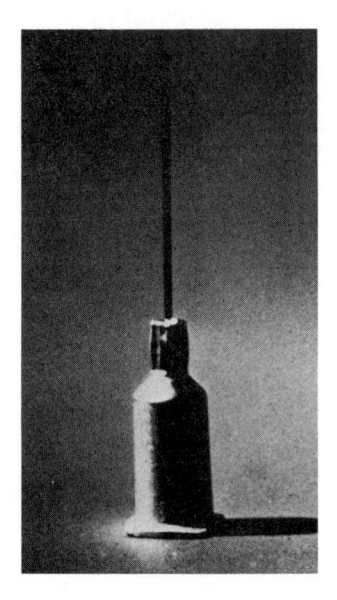

Figure 24. Disposable hypodermic needle lubricated with silicone fluid. The use of medical grade silicone fluid lubricants minimize pain and permit needles to be inserted and withdrawn from tissue with minimal force and without breakage or bending.

6. FRISCH   *Silicones in Artificial Organs*

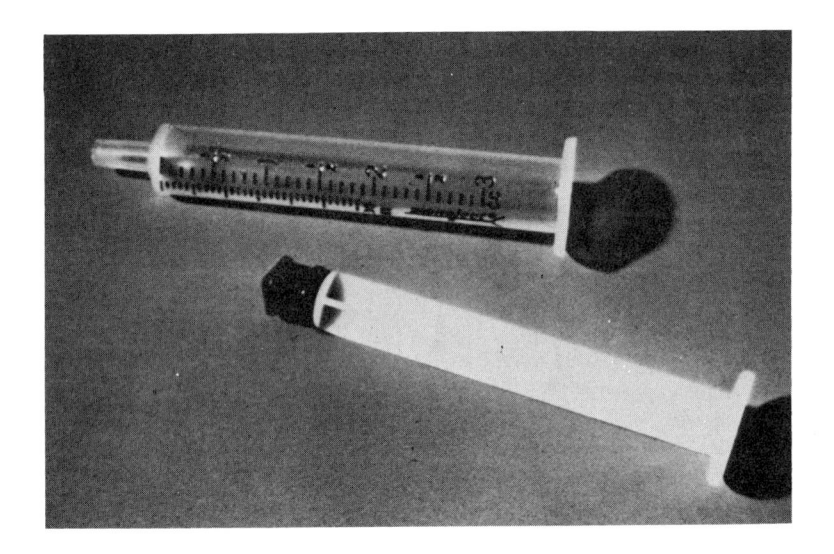

Figure 25. Disposable hypodermic syringe was made possible by the availability of medical grade silicone fluid to lubricate the plunger. Without an appropriate lubricant it would be essentially impossible to move the plunger tip inside the molded plastic barrel. Silicone fluid does not deteriorate with time, thus syringes may be stored for long periods of time without change in the forces required to move the plunger within the barrel.

quantities silicone fluids elicit no adverse effect, even with patients who must receive injections frequently such as those suffering from diabetes.

DISCUSSION AND CONCLUSIONS

Artificial organs and implants to replace diseased, defective, or destroyed components of the body are used by essentially every medical specialty. Medical grade silicone elastomer is the only elastomer generally recognized as safe and effective as a material of construction for soft, flexible, elastomeric implants. Carefully controlled formulations have been qualified by chronic biocompatibility and biodurability studies to provide a soft, flexible, elastomeric material of construction to meet many of the needs in these applications.

Literature Cited

1. F. S. Kipping, "Organic derivatives of silicon, Part II: The synthesis of benzylethylpropylsilicol, its sulfonation, and resolution of the D-L sulfonic derivatives into its optically active components", J. Chem. Soc. 91:209-240, 1907.
2. V. K. Rowe, H. C. Spencer, and S. L. Bass, "Toxicological studies on certain commercial silicones", J. Indust. Hyg. Tox. 30(6):332-352, Nov. 1948.
3. V. K. Rowe, H. C. Spencer, and S. L. Bass, "Toxicologic studies on certain commercial silicones", Arch. Indust. Hyg. Occup. Med. 1:539-544, May 1950.
4. J. Holter, "A father's last-chance invention saves his son", Reprint from The Reader's Digest, Jan. 1957.
5. R. E. Wilsnack, "Quantitative cell culture biocompatibility testing of medical devices and correlation to animal tests", Biomater. Med. Devices Artif. Organs 4(3 & 4):235-261, 1976.
6. R. E. Wilsnack, F. S. Meyer, and J. G. Smith, "Human cell culture toxicity testing of medical devices and correlation to animal tests", Biomater. Med. Devices Artif. Organs 1(3):543-562, 1973.
7. ASTM F748, "Recommended Practices for Selecting Generic Biological Test Methods for Materials and Devices", ASTM Standards for Medical and Surgical Materials and Devices.
8. J. W. Swanson and J. E. LeBeau, "The effect of implantation on the physical properties of silicone rubber", J. Biomed. Mater. Res. 8:357-367, 1974.
9. A. B. Swanson, "Flexible implant resection arthroplasty in the hand and extremities, The C. V. Mosby Co., St. Louis, 1973.
10. H. A. Lincoff, I. Baras, and J. McLean, "Modifications of the Custodis procedure for retinal detachment", Arch. Ophthalmol. 73:160-163, 1965.

11. J. Safian, "Progress in nasal and chin augmentation", Plast. Reconstr. Surg. 7:446-452, 1966.
12. G. B. Snyder, E. H. Courtiss, B. M. Kaye, and G. P. Gradinger, "A new chin implant for microgenia", Plast. Reconstr. Surg. 61:854-860, 1978.
13. T. D. Cronin, "Use of a Silastic® frame for total and subtotal reconstruction of the external ear: preliminary report", Plast. Reconstr. Surg. 37(5):399-405, May 1966.
14. T. D. Cronin and F. J. Gerow, "Augmentation mammaplasty: a new 'natural feel' prosthesis", Excerpta Medica International Congress, Series No. 66, Proceedings of the Third International Congress of Plastic Surgery, Washington, D.C., pp. 41-49, Oct. 1963.
15. C. H. Hine, H. W. Elliott, R. R. Wright, R. D. Cavalli, and C. D. Porter, "Evaluation of a Silicone Lubricant Injected Spinally", Toxicol. Appl. Pharmacol. 15, 566-573 (1969).

RECEIVED March 19, 1984

Characteristics of an Implantable Elastomer
Finger Joint Prosthesis Application

H. B. LEE, H. QUACH, D. B. BERRY, and W. J. STITH

Lord Corporation, Bioengineering Department, Erie, PA 16514

> Bion elastomer has been implanted in humans as part of the Biomeric finger joint prosthesis for the past four years. Clinical trial experience of the Biomeric prosthesis (over 500 joints implanted) in many research institutions has indicated that Bion elastomer has excellent stability, functionality, and biocompatibility. No adverse reactions to the material have been reported. Marketing approval for the prosthesis has been granted by the FDA. Extensive characterization of the basic polymer and its compounded elastomer, Bion, has been done to support its use as an implantable material suitable for a variety of medical applications. The material exhibits excellent biocompatibility, is resistant to oxidation, and is stable to irradiation at sterilization dose levels. Other major advantages are its high flex life and its low permeability by liquids. Physical properties can be tailored by judicious selection of polymer composition and elastomer formulation.

Since the mid-1950's, a number of finger prostheses have been developed for restoring function, correcting deformities, and relieving pain. Presently the leading products on the market are the Swanson and Niebauer prostheses (Figure 1).

In early 1960, Swanson (1) introduced the use of silicon rubber in this application. A cruciform bar of Silastic provided support across the joint and held the raw bone ends apart as a spacer. The major reported deficiencies of Swanson's product were fracture in the stem and the lack of stability in the joint cavity.

The Niebauer joint (2) is made of a Dacron-reinforced silicon rubber. The stems are covered with a Dacron mesh into which fibrous tissue can grow, thus effectively locking the stem in place. Its major deficiency is fracture across the hinge.

Beckenbaugh (3) reported that the fracture rates of Swanson

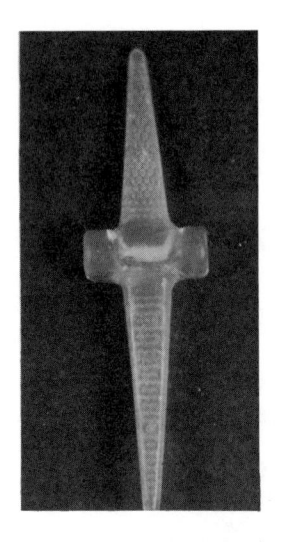

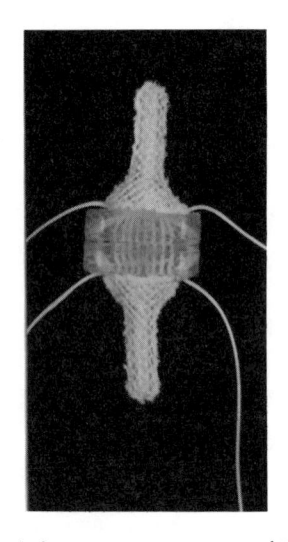

(A) Swanson joint (Dow Corning)   (B) Niebauer joint (Sutter)

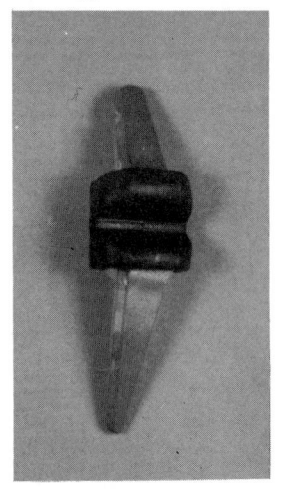

(C) Biomeric joint (Lord Corporation)

Figure 1. Finger prosthesis.

and Niebauer prostheses, with an average follow-up of two and one-half years in clinical investigation, were 26.2% and 38.2%, respectively.

In the early 1970's, Lord Corporation began to look toward the orthopaedic field as a natural extension of its expertise in elastomeric bearings. The elastomeric bearing principle applied to prostheses imparts stability and controlled motion without incurring high restraining forces. The use of elastomer allowed the joint design to consist of titanium stems for fixation, a pin positioned transversely through the elastomeric section for lateral stability, and an elastomer bridge bonded between the titanium stems.

Selection of Elastomer

Numerous elastomers were evaluated for finger joint prosthesis application. Hexsyn showed the best characteristics for this application.

For several years, Goodyear supplied their compounded polymer under the name of Hexsyn to various research centers; namely, Monsanto Research Corporation (4), Washington University (5), National Bureau of Standards (6), Cleveland Clinic (7), and Thermoelectron Corporation (8). These institutions have research programs for physical testing of polymers for use in circulatory assist devices and for the development and evaluation of a cardiac prosthesis funded by the NHLB-NIH.

The objective of the first three institutions' projects is to develop short-term fatigue test methodologies that will predict long-term *in vitro* performance of elastomers used in the devices and to evaluate the fatigue life of candidate materials for potential use in the devices. Cleveland Clinic and Thermoelectron Corporation utilize this elastomer for pumping diaphragms.

Flex Life. Kiraly and Hillegass (9) reported flex life of various polymers as shown in Table I. Their results show clearly that the flex life of Hexsyn is superior to that of other elastomers.

Poirier (10) at Thermoelectron Corporation investigated seven elastomers for blood pump bladder applications. The flex life of diaphragms from the elastomers showed that Hexsyn, Pellethane, and Biomer were significantly superior to Tecoflex HR, Tecothane B, Silastic, and SRI.

McMillin (11) at Monsanto investigated uniaxial fatigue life of various elastomers in air, nitrogen, oxygen, saline, and blood environments. His method of accelerating fatigue indicated cut-initiated fatigue testing to be significant in predicting long-term, low strain fatigue failure. In this respect, Hexsyn rubber was ranked number one among the test materials.

Table I. Flex Life of Various Polymers
ASTM D430 DeMattia Test Machine

Polymer	Cycles to Failure (millions)
Silicone rubber	0.8
styrene-butadiene rubber	4
natural rubber	4
oxypropylene rubber	10
ethylene-propylenediene-terpolymer	15
Biomer	18
Hexsyn	352 (no failure)

Biocompatibility. Primary acute toxicity screening tests of the elastomer were conducted by Materials Science Toxicology Laboratories at the University of Tennessee, Johnson & Johnson Research Foundation, and North American Science Association using standard procedures.

Results of primary acute toxicity screening tests on medical grade Hexsyn elastomer are summarized in Table II and show excellent biocompatibility of the material and its extracts.

Table II. Biocompatibility Testing of Hexsyn

Tests Directly on Sample:

Tissue Culture--Agar Overlay	Non-cytotoxic
Intramuscular Implant (Rat)	Non-toxic
Intracutaneous Implant (Rat)	Non-toxic
Hemolysis Test	Not significant

Tests on Extracts:

Tissue Culture--MEM Elution	Non-cytotoxic
Intracutaneous Test (Rabbits)	Non-irritating
Systemic Toxicity (Mice)	No adverse effects
Cell Growth Inhibition	Not significant
Ames Mutagenicity Test	Non-mutagenic

Implantable Bion Elastomer

In 1979, Lord Corporation became the sole supplier of Hexsyn rubber under license from Goodyear Tire and Rubber Company. Minor changes were made in the polymerization process of the basic polymer to compensate for larger scale production runs, and the original elastomer formulation was modified by slightly reducing the levels of cure agents and sulfur. The new formulation, known as Bion, maintained physical properties and enhanced biocompatibility.

Composition. Bion polymer is a terpolymer of 1-hexene and 4-methyl-1,4-hexadiene and 5-methyl-1,4-hexadiene, the crosslinking agent. The polymer is compounded with carbon black and traditional vulcanization aides. A standard formulation contains 3 mol % crosslinking agent (% relative to 1-hexene) and 50 phr carbon black loading. Elastomer for implantation use is extracted with an appropriate solvent in a Soxhlet-type extractor to remove by-products of vulcanization and any leachable material.

Polymer Properties. Physical characteristics of the basic polymer are summarized in Table III.

Table III. Characteristics of Bion Polymer

Molecular weight:	$M_n = 0.6 - 1.0 \times 10^6$
Molecular weight distribution:	$M_w/M_n = 1.5 - 1.8$
Gel content:	Less than 3%
Residual solvent:	Less than 2%
Color:	White

Dilute solution viscosity measurements were made using a Cannon-Fenske viscometer. Number average molecular weight (Mn) and weight average molecular weight (Mw) were calculated from viscosity measurements and the Mark-Houwink Constants (12). Gel content was determined by a modification of procedure ASTM D3616.

Elastomer Properties. Mechanical properties, wettability, and swelling characteristics of a typical elastomer are summarized in Table IV.

Table IV. Characteristics of Bion Elastomer

Flex life (ASTM D430):	over 300×10^6 cycles
Tensile strength:	13.1 MPa
Elongation at breaking point:	350%
Tear strength (ASTM D624, Die C):	24.5 KN/M
Contact angle of water:	$1/2(\theta rec + \theta adv) = 50°$
Swelling in hexane at room temperature:	170 wt. %
Swelling in H$_2$O at 37°C:	0.9 wt. %

Flex life, a measure of rubber deterioration by dynamic fatigue, was determined on a DeMattia flexing machine (ASTM D430). Tensile and tear properties were determined on elastomer sheets (1/8 inch thick) using ASTM D412 and ASTM D624 respectively. The contact angle of water on the elastomer was measured with a captive air bubble method (13).

Resistance to Irradiation. Since medical devices are often sterilized by gamma-radiation, material properties must be maintained after irradiation.

Physical properties of the Bion elastomer were measured following irradiation of one, three, and five times the standard sterilization dose level (2.5 Mrads). Tensile strength did not change significantly up to 12.7 Mrads irradiation. Elongation and swellability decreased while hardness increased with dosage due to increased crosslink density in the rubber. The loss of low molecular weight polymer by extraction increased slightly (Table V).

Table V. Radiation Effects on Bion Elastomer

(Tensile Properties)

Dose (Mrads)	100% Modulus (MPa)	300% Modulus (MPa)	Ultimate Tensile (MPa)	Ultimate Elong. (%)
0	1.5	8.3	13.1	430
2.5	1.8	9.4	13.1	390
7.6	2.0	9.7	11.7	350
12.7	2.2	10.7	12.4	350

(Hardness, Extractables, and Swelling)

Dose (Mrads)	Hardness Shore A	Extractable %	Swelling in hexane Wt. Gain (%)
0	61+1	1.0	168+3
2.5	63+1	2.0	156+4
7.6	63+1	2.4	150+2
12.7	65+1	2.9	147+2

Permeability. Bion elastomer has much less diffusion of silicon oil and water than silicon rubber under the same testing conditions (ASTM D814). Comparative permeation rates are listed on Table VI. Applications demanding low permeable materials include implantation of encapsulated electronic devices and silicon oil-filled breast prostheses.

Table VI. Permeation Rate of Silicon Oil and Water

Membrane	Diffusate	Permeation Rate gm/in^2 day
Bion	Silicon oil (a)	0.08 x 10^{-2} (b)
Silastic (a)	Silicon oil (a)	0.8 x 10^{-2} (b)
Bion	H$_2$O	0.01 (c)
Silastic (a)	H$_2$O	0.2 (c)

(a): materials for breast implant supplied by Medical Engineering
(b): under vacuum at 37°C
(c): under forced air oven at 37°C

Dispersion. The degree of filler dispersion is very important in obtaining reproducible and desirable characteristics of any filled rubber. The advantage of fine particle fillers is lost if aggregates of particles are not broken down and if the particles are not well distributed throughout the elastomer. Therefore, all elastomers are evaluated for homogeneity of dispersion before being accepted for testing and use.

A simple qualitative visual method for rating the dispersion of fillers (50phr carbon black) in Bion elastomer was developed and is illustrated in Figure 2. A cross section of cured elastomer is examined under a binocular microscope to check gross dispersion of fillers. The visual dispersion is rated against a set of standard photographs of dispersions which had previously been ranked and correlated with certain important physical properties. For example, in Figure 3, the flex life of a well dispersed elastomer was over 300 million cycles while that of a poorly dispersed one was below one million cycles. The correlation of physical properties to dispersion has been substantiated with other rubbers (14).

Effect of Crosslinker Content

A wide variety of physical properties of Bion elastomer can be obtained through variation of crosslinker amounts in the raw polymer and of carbon black levels in the compounded elastomer.

Figure 3 shows typical rheometer cure time curves of three Bion elastomers with different crosslinker levels at 50 phr carbon black loading. With higher crosslinker content in the polymer, the torque required to shear the rubber during vulcanization increased while cure time decreased.

A typical cure time of compounded elastomer having 50 phr carbon black and 3% crosslinker in the raw polymer is 48 minutes

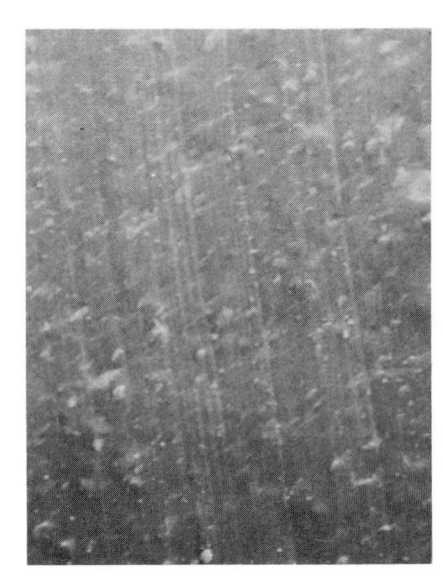

(A) Good dispersion   (B) Poor dispersion

Figure 2. Comparison of filler dispersion.

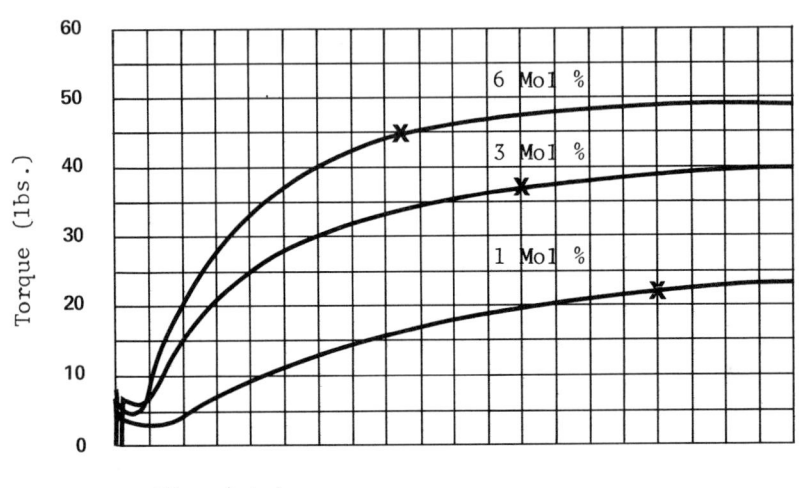

Figure 3. Effect of cross-linker level on cure characteristics. (Monsanto rheometer curves - 307 °F)

Table VII. Cure Time and Flex Life of Various Bion Elastomers

Crosslinker Mole %	Carbon Black (phr)	Cure Time (min.)	Flex Life (cycles)
1	50	64	not determined
1	65	66	not determined
1	80	68	not determined
3	35	46	not determined
3	50	48	over 300×10^6 (no failure)
3	80	50	over 8×10^6 (no failure)
3	100	50	3×10^6 (failure)

at 307°F; material containing 1% crosslinker has a substantially longer cure time of 68 minutes (Table VII).

Physical properties of various Bion elastomers with variation of crosslinker amounts in the raw polymer and carbon black levels in the compounded elastomer are summarized in Table VIII.

Overall, as crosslinker content increased, cure time substantially decreased. As crosslinker content increases, modulus and hardness increase but ultimate tensile strength, elongation and swelling decrease. Permeability to water was unchanged.

Effect of Carbon Black Loading

Unlike crosslinker content, the level of carbon black in the elastomer did not significantly affect cure time (Table VII) but did have a dramatic effect upon flex fatigue life. In order to obtain high flex life, the maximum loading of carbon black was limited to 80 phr.

Tear resistance, modulus, and hardness increase along with the filler content.

Material characteristics can be tailored to suit a desired application. For example, blood compatibility of various Bion elastomers was investigated in the atria of goats by Dr. Williams' group (15) in Toronto. Initial results indicated that elastomers containing high levels of carbon black showed greater thrombo resistance than those with lower amounts or no carbon black.

Conclusion

Bion elastomer is an implantable material suitable for a variety of medical applications. The material exhibits excellent biocompatibility, is resistant to oxidation, and is stable to irradiation at sterilization dose levels. Major advantages are its high

Table VIII. Physical Properties of Various Bion Elastomers

Crosslinker Mole % (a)	Carbon Black (phr) (b)	100% Modulus (MPa)	300% Modulus (MPa)	Ultimate Tensile (MPa)	Ultimate Elongation (%)	Water Diffusion (mg/day cm^2)	Hardness (Shore A)	Tear Resist. KN/M	Swelling Hexane % Wt. Increase
1	50	1.2	0.6	17.0	612	1.9	53	24	218
1	65	1.4	7.1	16.0	580	1.9	61	26	184
1	80	2.0	8.4	14.4	496	1.6	63	30	N/A
3	0	0.2	N/A	1.4	267	2.3	24	1	375
3	35	1.7	9.7	12.7	364	1.7	54	14	193
3	50	2.2	10.1	15.0	412	1.9	61	25	161
3	65	2.7	12.7	16.7	353	1.6	69	27	134
3	80	2.9	13.5	16.6	381	1.7	78	28	104
6	0	0.4	N/A	1.0	187	2.0	29	4	N/A
6	50	3.6	N/A	11.8	235	1.9	68	23	129

a: Initial feed amount during polymerization
b: Parts per 100 parts raw polymer
N/A: Not available

NOTE: Tensile, tear, hardness, and flex life characteristics were determined with ASTM D412, D2240, D624, and D430, respectively. Cure time was determined with a Monsanto rheometer, Model R-100. Swelling characteristics of the elastomer were measured by weight difference after soaking the square shape (1 x 1 x 0.2 cm) in hexane for 28 hours at room temperature.

flex life and its low permeability by liquids. Physical properties can be tailored by judicious selection of polymer composition and elastomer formulation.

Bion elastomer has been implanted in humans as part of the Biomeric finger joint prosthesis for the past four years.

Literature Cited

1. Swanson, A. B., J. Bone Joint Surg., 1972, 54A, 435.
2. Niebauer, J. J., J. Bone Joint Surg., 1968, 50A, 634.
3. Beckenbaugh, R. D., Dobyns, J. H., Linscheid, R. L. and Bryan, R. S., J. Bone Joint Surg., 1976, 58A, 483.
4. McMillin, C. R., Orofino, T. A. and Sheppard, D. L., "Physical Testing of Polymers", Devices and Technology Branch Contractors Meeting Program, U.S. Department of Health, Education and Welfare, 1979, p. 80.
5. Kardos, J. L., Sanson, W. M. and Clark, R. E., "Physical Testing of Polymers for Use in Circulatory Assist Devices", Devices and Technology Branch Contractors Meeting Program, U.S. Department of Health, Education and Welfare, 1979, p.81.
6. Penn, R. W. and McKenna G. B., "Physical Testing of Polymer for Use in Circulatory Assist Devices", Devices and Technology Branch Contractors Meeting Program, U.S. Department of Health, Education and Welfare, 1979, p. 83.
7. Nose, Y., et al., "Development and Evaluation of Cardiac Prostheses", Annual Report, NIH-NHLB N01-HV-4-2960-5, Cleveland Clinic Foundation, Cleveland, Ohio, 1979.
8. Poirier, V., "Fabrication of Cardiovascular Devices", Devices and Technology Branch Contractors Meeting Program, U.S. Department of Health, Education and Welfare, 1979, p. 35.
9. Kiraly, R. J. and Hillegass, D. V., "Polyolefin Blood Pump Components in Synthetic Biomedical Polymers: Concept and Applications", Szycher, M., Robinson W. J., Eds., Technomic Publishing Company, Inc.: Westport, 1980, p. 59.
10. Poirier, V., "Fabrication and Testing of Flocked Blood Bladders in Synthetic Biomedical Polymers: Concepts and Applications", Szycher M., Robinson, W. J., Eds., Technomic Publishing Company, Inc.: Westport, 1980, p. 73.
11. McMillin, C. R., "Physical Testing of Polymers for Use in Circulatory Assist Devices", Annual Report, NIH-NHLB N01-HV-7-2918-3, Monsanto Research Corporation, Dayton, Ohio, 1980.
12. Lin, F. C., Stivala, S. S. and Biesenberger, J. A., J. Appl. Polym. Sci., 1973, 17, 1073.
13. Andrade, et al., J. Polym. Sci.: Polym. Symp., 1979, 66, 313.
14. Morton, M., Rubber Technology, Van Nostrand Reinhold Company: New York, 1973, Chapter 3.
15. Williams, W. G., Hospital for Sick Children, Toronto, personal communication.

RECEIVED March 19, 1984

The Current Status of Prosthetic Heart Valves

AJIT P. YOGANATHAN, E. C. HARRISON, and R. H. FRANCH

Bio Fluid Dynamics Laboratory, School of Chemical Engineering, Georgia Institute of Technology, Atlanta, GA 30332

The main objective of the study is to correlate the in vitro fluid dynamic performances of prosthetic heart valves with their in vivo clinical and pathological characteristics. The aim is to clearly document any relationships between in vitro fluid dynamic performance and potential clinical and/or pathological findings and complications. Heart valve prostheses have been used successfully since 1960. Of the nearly 50 different cardiac valves introduced over the past 22 years, many have been discarded due to their lack of success, and of those remaining, several modifications have been made. The most commonly used basic types of prosthetic valves are: (a) caged ball, (b) tilting disc, (c) caged disc, (d) bi-leaflet and (e) bioprostheses. The most serious problems and complications associated with valve prostheses are: (a) thromboembolism, (b) tissue overgrowth, (c) infection, (d) tearing of sewing sutures, (e) hemolysis, (f) valve failure due to material fatigue or chemical change, (g) damage to the endothelial tissue lining of the vessel wall adjacent to the valve, (h) large pressure gradients especially under exercise conditions, and (i) excess regurgitation. Problems (a), (b), (e), (g) - (i) are directly related to the fluid dynamics associated with the different prosthetic valve designs, and are discussed in detail in this paper.

Heart valve prostheses have been used successfully since 1960. As stated by Roberts ([1]) the decade of 1960 will probably be remembered most in the annals of cardiology as the decade during which cardiac valve replacement became a successful reality. Of the nearly 50 different cardiac valves introduced over the past 22 years, many have been discarded due to their lack of success, and of those remaining, several modifications have been made or are being made at the time of this writing. The most commonly used basic types of prosthetic valves at present are (a) caged ball, (b) tilting disc, (c) caged disc, (d) bi-leaflet and (e) bioprostheses. At present over 75,000 prosthetic valves of different designs are used annually throughout the world. Even after 20 years of experience the problems associated with heart valve prostheses have not been totally eliminated. The most serious problems and complications associated with heart valve prostheses are: (a) thromboembolism, (b) tissue overgrowth, (c) infection, (d) tearing of sewing sutures, (e) red cell destruction (hemolysis), (f) valve failure due to material fatigue or chemical change, (g) damage to the endothelial tissue lining of the vessel wall adjacent to the valve and (h) leaks caused by failure of the valve to close properly. Problems (a), (b), (e) and (g) are <u>directly</u> related to the fluid dynamics associated with the various prosthetic heart valves, and need to be addressed in more detail by investigators studying bio-fluid mechanics. The other problems are indirectly related to the fluid mechanics. The problems relating to valve failure due to material fatigue or chemical change also need to be studied especially as they relate to bioprostheses.

Tissue bioprostheses gained widespread use during the mid-1970's. It was even naively thought by some of the tissue valve manufacturers that the ideal heart valve prosthesis had been discovered. The major advantage of tissue bioprostheses compared to their mechanical counterparts is that they have a lower incidence of thromboembolic complications. Therefore, tissue valves for a large part can be used without anticoagulation therapy to eliminate or reduce thromboembolic complications. Unfortunately, the tissue bioprostheses clinically used at present also have major disadvantages such as: (a) relatively large pressure drops compared to some of the mechanical valves, especially in the smaller sizes, (b) jet-like flow through the valve leaflets, (c) material fatigue and/or wear of valve leaflets, (d) calcification of valve leaflets, especially in children and young adults. Because of these and other drawbacks, valve manufacturers are now developing new designs of mechanical valves such as the St. Jude, Hall-Kaster and Omni-Science prostheses, newer designs of bioprostheses and trileaflet valves made from polymeric materials.

The ideal heart valve prosthesis has not yet been designed and probably will never exist. An ideal valve should have the following characteristics:
1. Be fully sterile at the time of implantation and be nontoxic.
2. Be surgically convenient to insert at or near the normal location in the heart.
3. Conform to the heart structure rather than the heart structure conforming to the valve (i.e., the size and shape of the prosthesis should not interfere with cardiac function).

4. Show a minimum resistance to flow so as to prevent a significant pressure drop across the valve.
5. Have minimal reverse flow necessary for valve closure, so as to keep the incompetence of the valve at a low level.
6. Show long mechanical and structural wear of the valve.
7. Be long-lasting (∼ 25 years), and maintain its normal functional performance (i.e., must not deteriorate with time).
8. Cause minimum trauma to blood elements and the endothelial tissue of the cardiovascular structure surrounding the valve.
9. Show a low probability for thromboembolic complications without the use of anticoagulants.
10. Should not be noisy and disturb the patient.
11. Should be radiographically visible.
12. Should have a modest price.

As stated previously the serious problems of thromboembolism, excess tissue overgrowth, red-cell and platelet damage, and damage to the endothelial lining of the vessel wall adjacent to the valve are directly related to the fluid dynamics associated with the various types of valve prostheses. Blackshear and his co-workers (2,3) suggest that the shear stresses required in the bulk of the flow to hemolyze red blood cells are about 40,000 dynes/cm^2. Nevaril and his co-workers (4) contend, however, that this value could be as low as 1500 dynes/cm^2. In vitro experiments (5-7) have also recently shown that platelets could be damaged by shear stresses of the order of 100 - 500 dynes/cm^2. A formed element such as a red blood cell which adheres to the vessel wall or to a foreign surface (such as the valve super-structure) may be damaged by shear stresses of the order of 10-10^2 dynes/cm^2 (2,3,8). Lloyd et al., (9) indicate that sublethal damage to red blood cells could occur at shear stresses on the order of 500 dynes/cm^2 or less. A recent study by McIntyre (10) indicates that the red blood cells of heart valve patients are more filterable in micropores than compared to normal subjects, due to sublethal damage to the red cells of valve recipients. Lethal damage to red blood cells causes hemolysis which in turn leads to anemia. Sublethal and/or lethal damage to red blood cells could also lead to platelet adhesion, aggregation and coagulation, resulting in thrombus formation. Mechanical damage to platelets (lethal and sublethal) will eventually lead to thromboembolic complications.

Fry (11,12) has conducted two studies on the effects of wall shear on the endothelial lining of the aortic wall. He found that the endothelial cells on the vessel wall could be damaged at wall-shear stresses of about 400 dynes/cm^2 and could be eroded off the vessel wall at shear stresses of about 950 dynes/cm^2. He observed that when the endothelial surface was exposed to shearing stresses above some critical value (400 dynes/cm^2) the cells began to suffer structural and chemical changes. The critical stress is known as the "yielding" stress.

If a shearing stress above the critical value is applied for a long time period, the yielding process continues until the cells become mechanically unstable and are washed away from their moorings to the basement membrane in total or by progressive erosion of cell substance. As the eroded surface of the vessel wall is exposed to the flowing blood, deposition of blood elements and thrombotic materials occur. Fry found that the deposited material consisted of fibrous tissue, platelets, red blood cells, and other unidentified debris. He states that such deposition could lead to intimal thickening of the vessel wall. Woolf and Carstairs (13) state that the fibrous tissue observed on the aortic wall as a result of intiamal thickening owes its presence to either infiltration or thrombus formation, or a combination of these two factors.

Platelets do not adhere to intact endothelial cells but they do adhere to subendothelial connective tissue composed of collagen and other materials. Platelets, however, have access to collagen fibers once the endothelial lining of a vessel wall is damaged or eroded off. The adhesion of platelets to the damaged vessel leads to the subsequent release of ADP and platelet factor 3 (PF-3). These substances play an active role in platelet aggregation and coagulation, respectively, and may lead to thrombus formation. A red blood cell will not stick to the intact endothelial lining of a vessel wall. If, however, the vessel intima is damaged resulting in a loss of endothelial integrity, red blood cells could adhere onto the vessel wall. If the adhered red blood cell is exposed to shears on the order of 10 to 100 dynes/cm^2 it will probably be lethally damaged and hemolyzed. Red blood cells contain ADP and a clot-promoting factor known as erythrocin. These substances are released into the plasma as a result of hemolysis, initiating both platelet aggregation and coagulation, which in turn may lead to thrombus formation.

The mechanical damage to the blood elements, as well as to the endothelial tissue of the adjacent vessel wall, may in addition trigger the complex biochemical reactions which could lead to the excess fibrous tissue overgrowth observed on some recovered heart valves. Therefore, large wall and bulk turbulent shear stresses could cause serious problems and complications in vivo.

It is also well known that regions of flow stagnation, flow separation and excessively low shear, in the immediate vicinity of the valve superstructure have been related to thrombus formation and/or excess tissue overgrowth on the prosthesis. The flow velocity, shear stress and pressure fields in the immediate vicinity of a given heart valve prosthesis design are directly related to the fluid dynamic characteristics of the prosthesis. Therefore, detailed in vitro fluid dynamic studies should help predict potential problems and complications that may arise in vivo with different designs of prosthetic heart valves.

Methodology

An extensive study of the literature was undertaken, and results from over 450 articles in both the medical and engineering literature were utilized (14). The results for the following heart valve prostheses are summarized in this paper: (a) Starr-Edwards ball valves, (b) Kay-Shiley disc valve, (c) Beall disc valve, (d) Bjork-Shiley tilting disc valve, (e) Hancock porcine valve, and (f) St. Jude bi-leaflet valve. These valve prostheses shown in Figures 1 through 6 were chosen because of their past and/or present popularity in clinical use. They also encompass all the basic designs of valve prostheses used during the past two decades.

In vivo pressure drop, in vitro pressure drop and regurgitation (reflux and leakage), hemolysis, and thromboembolic complication (TEC) data were obtained and tabulated for each of the above valves. The in vitro pressure drop results were obtained in most instances from pulsatile flow measurements. The in vivo pressure drop results presented focus primarily on patients who were electively catheterized and who did not have any clinical problems related to the prosthesis. The results should therefore reflect the in vivo hemodynamic performance of normally functioning prostheses. Valve areas (VA), or otherwise known as the effective orifice areas, were calculated by the various investigators from the Gorlin or modified Gorlin formulae (15). The in vivo valve areas give a good qualitative and/or quantitative ranking for the in vivo pressure drop characteristics of the various valves. If different valve designs are studied by the same investigators and/or at the same medical center, the results have more quantitative significance. Even though the absolute values of VA may vary from center to center for a given valve design, the ranking of different valve types according to in vivo valve areas are generally consistent. The main reasons for the variations in the absolute values from center to center are: (i) inaccuracies in obtaining cardiac catheterization data (pressures and flows), (ii) obtaining a statistically large enough patient population and (iii) different formulae used to estimate VA. The in vivo results do not contain regurgitation data because this parameter cannot be quantitatively measured during catheterization, or other in vivo procedures, at the present time.

In vitro pressure drop, flow rate, and regurgitation data were in most cases obtained directly from their respective articles. From these data the valve areas (VA) (i.e.: effective orifice area) were calculated from the following formula:

$$VA\ (cm^2) = \frac{Q_{rms}}{51.6\ \sqrt{\overline{\Delta p}}}$$

where
  Q_{rms} = root mean square systolic or diastolic flow rate, cm^3/s
  $\Delta \bar{p}$ = mean systolic or diastolic pressure drop, mmHg

In vitro regurgitation volume (RV) data in the bio-medical engineering literature is generally poorly reported. Only RV data expressed in cm^3/stroke or data that could be calculated (from the information provided) into such a form were used. In many instances, RV would be expressed in the literature as a percentage, with no information on cardiac output and/or heart rate. The work of Dellsperger et al., (16) and in our laboratory tend to indicate that for a given valve, at a fixed heart rate the value of RV in cm^3/stroke does not vary (except within experimental error) with cardiac output.

The in vitro pressure drop and regurgitation results give a very good qualitative and/or quantitative ranking of the stenotic and regurgitant characteristics of the various valve designs. If different valve types were studied by the same investigator the results obtained will have more quantitative importance. Even though the absolute numerical values obtained by different investigators may vary for a given valve design, the ranking of the different valve types are generally consistent. The major reasons for the variations in the absolute values among the different investigators is because different types of pulse duplicators and flow chamber geometries have been used. It should, however, be noted that there is better quantitative agreement in the in vitro pressure drop and regurgitation data between different investigators, than with the in vivo hemodynamic data from different medical centers.

Information obtained from the in vitro flow visualization, and velocity and shear stress measurement studies will be discussed in the text.

All the hemolysis and thromboembolic complication (TEC) tables were constructed from information extracted from their respective articles. During the study it was noticed that there is no consistent scientific manner in which data on hemolysis and TEC's are reported in the medical literature. Elevated LDH levels, and reduced and/or absent haptaglobin levels are good indicators of intravascular hemolysis. Reduced half-lifes of red cells and platelets are in our opinion one of the best ways of monitoring mechanical (shear) damage to blood elements. Such tests are infrequently done in a clinical environment. Early TEC's and deaths are defined as those occurring during the first 30 days after valve replacement surgery. TEC events are expressed where possible as patient ratios and/or as a rate (% per pt. yr.).

Based on the hemolysis and TEC data and other pertinent information in the literature, we have been able to draw certain conclusions about the hemolytic and thromboembolic potential of the different valve designs. The locations of thrombus formation, excess tissue growth and related valve dysfunctions will be discussed in the text.

Results and Discussion

(1) Starr Edwards Ball Valves
(a) Valve Description

The Starr-Edwards 1200/1260 Aortic and 6120 Mitral prostheses are closed single-cage Silastic ball valves. They are comprised of a radio-opaque polished Stellite alloy No. 21 cage with a sewing ring which combines Teflon (TFE-fluorocarbon) and polypropylene cloth. The Model 1260 and 6120 poppets contain 2-percent-by-weight barium sulfate for radiopacity as do some of the 1200 occluders. The model 1200 aortic valve was made available in January 1966. It was superseded in 1968 by the model 1260. The cloth was extended slightly further to the orifice in the model 1260 valve to resemble the cloth metal interface of the model 6120 mitral prosthesis. The model 6120 mitral valve has a four strut cage to distinguish it from the aortic valves which have 3 strut cages.

The model 2310/2320 (aortic) and 6310/6320 (mitral) Starr-Edwards valves evolved from the totally Dacron cloth-covered models 2300 aortic and 6300 mitral metallic ball valve prostheses. The totally cloth covered valves were available from 1967 to 1968. They were discontinued primarily because of a problem of excessive overgrowth of autogenous tissue in the flow orifice and a problem of orifice cloth durability. The first series (models 2310/6310) of Starr-Edwards composite seat valves became available in 1968. They were comprised of a Teflon/Polypropylene cloth-covered Stellite No. 21 cage with exposed metal supports in the orifice which formed a composite seat against which the ball could close. The composite seat design increased the orifice area by approximately 15% and the orifice-to-ball diameter from about 86% to 90%. It also reduced somewhat the problem of orifice cloth wear. Unfortunately, the close clearance between ball and cage-struts of the model 2310 allowed small amounts of autogenous tissue to interfere with motion of the ball. In 1970, models 2320/6320 were introduced, and models 2310/6310 were discontinued. For all due purposes, model 2320 was a duplicate of model 2310 except for an increase in ball-strut clearance. Although changes were also made in the fabric of the 2320/6320 models, cloth wear and tissue overgrowth continued to be major problems. These problems eventually led to the discontinuance of these models in 1976.

Models 2400 (aortic) and 6400 (mitral) Starr-Edwards composite track valve prostheses are closed single-cage hollow metallic ball valve prostheses. The cage struts, poppets, and metallic closure supports on the inner aspect of the base ring are made of Haynes alloy No. 21 (Stellite alloy No. 21) and are easily seen radiographically. The inner aspect of the cage struts has no cloth covering and hence no metal-cloth contact. The rest of the cage struts are covered by tubular-knitted porous polypropylene cloth. The orifice cloth is made from siliconized multi-filament Dacron thread which together with

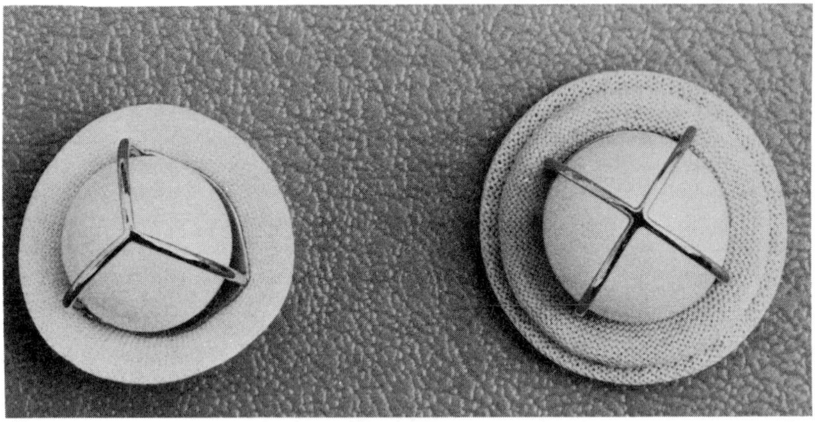

Figure 1. (a) Starr-Edwards ball valve, model 1260
(b) Starr-Edwards ball valve, model 6120

the exposed metallic supports produces a composite seating surface which the ball impacts at closure. The sewing ring is made of Teflon and polypropylene cloth over a silicone foam padding. The model 2400 valve has 3-strut cage while the model 6400 cage has 4 struts.

(b) <u>In Vivo</u> Results

The Starr-Edwards aortic ball valve prostheses had valve areas (VA's) of 0.92 to 1.9 cm^2, for valve sizes of 21 to 29 mm. For the mitral prostheses in the size range of 26 to 34 mm, VA's were in the range of 1.4 to 2.7 cm^2. These values are similar to those observed with other ball valve prostheses, such as the Smeloff valve design.

There are numerous articles on the hemolysis and thromboembolic complications created by the different designs of Starr-Edwards ball valves. The results indicate without a doubt that the completely cloth covered strut models 2300, 2310, 2320, 6300, 6310 and 6320 caused moderate and in many cases severe hemolysis (17-22). The models 2400 and 6400 tend to cause less hemolysis compared to the other cloth covered Starr-Edwards ball valves (18,23-25). The models 1200/1260 and 6120 non-cloth covered valves cause mild to moderate hemolysis. The thromboembolic complications seem to be greater with the non-cloth covered models (1200, 1260, 6000, 6120) compared to the cloth covered models (2300, 2310, 2320, 2400, 6300, 6310, 6320, 6400). This fact is substantiated in clinical studies conducted on both cloth and non-cloth covered models by the same group of researchers (18,26-30). According to Lefrak and Starr (31), the cloth covered valves have an embolus free rate of 95% at 3 years versus 81% for the non-cloth covered prostheses. The TEC rates for the Starr-Edwards ball valves seem to be in the range of 3 to 6.5% per pt. yr. with anticoagulation therapy and as high as 10% per pt. yr. without anticoagulation therapy. The cloth covered Starr-Edwards ball valves were developed in an attempt to reduce thromboembolic complications by encouraging a thin layer of endothelialization on the cloth covering. The cloth covered valves, however, do require anticoagulation therapy. This was determined quite conclusively from clinical studies where anticoagulation therapy was not used (18,32,33,34).

Thrombus formation and tissue overgrowth on various parts of the super structure of the Starr-Edwards ball valves is well documented (19,31-38). Roberts and his co-workers (18,35-37) give detailed pathologic descriptions of the thrombus formation and tissue overgrowth observed on Starr-Edwards ball valves. The examinations of recovered Starr-Edwards aortic and mitral ball valves have shown: (i) thrombus formation at the apex of the cage, at the base of the three struts and in varying degrees along the struts, and (ii) excess tissue growth on the downstream side of the sewing ring on all models, along the struts (inside and outside) and along the fabric on the inside surface of the orifice of the cloth covered models. Thrombus has also been observed on the inflow surface of the orifice ring. Studies by Roberts and his co-workers (1,19,35-37) have also observed endothelial damage and tissue proliferation of the proximal ascending aorta in patients with aortic prostheses.

They have found intimal thickening of the aortic root including the area of the coronary arterial ostia. The thickening was produced by the deposition of fibrous tissue on the internal elastic membrane of the proximal ascending aorta. The degree of intimal proliferation varied from minimal to extremely severe. In some cases the intimal thickening involved not only the ascending aorta but also the proximal coronary arteries. Roberts (1) states that intimal fibrosis in the aortic root may be a previously unrecognized consequence of aortic valve replacement, and is a potential problem with all peripheral flow type aortic prostheses.

The combination of thrombus formation and fibrous tissue overgrowth can be a lethal combination, as has been learned from the recovered Starr-Edwards ball valves. The idea of growing a thin layer of neo-intima along the fabric of the cloth covered valves did not uniformly succeed. With all the cloth covered models (2300-10-20, 2400, 6300-10-20, 6400), tissue overgrowth occurred on the fabric which lined the orifice and at times caused the valves to become stenotic. In addition, the models with the completely fabric covered cages (2300-10-20, 6300-10-20), could develop excessive fibrous tissue and thrombus growth on the inner aspects of the struts which could in turn cause: either (i) the poppet to stick in an open position, or (ii) a reduction in the opening excursion of the poppet. If the stuck poppet phenomena was not diagnosed immediately the consequences were generally fatal. The 2300-10-20 and 6300-10-20 models also had varying degrees of cloth wear due to abrasion between the metal poppet and the fabric. Cloth wear with these prostheses often led to severe hemolytic anemia. The models 2400 and 6400 do not seem to suffer from the problem of cloth wear and that is probably one of the reasons why they cause less hemolysis compared to the 2300 and 6300 series. They do, however, seem to cause more hemolysis compared to the non-cloth covered (1200/1260, 6120) prostheses. The fact that the cloth covered models caused more hemolysis compared to the non-cloth covered models is highlighted in studies where both types of valves were investigated (17-25).

Hamby et al., (39) in an excellent clinical study, demonstrated the hydrodynamic instability of the Starr-Edwards aortic ball valves in 41 patients. The study combined cinefluoroscopy, phonocardiography and hemodynamic measurements. In 20 of the patients the poppet remained in a relatively fixed position (even though it rotated) at the apex of the cage during systolic ejection. In 11 patients the poppet bounced away from the apex of the cage during early ejection and promptly returned to the apex during the remainder of the ejection period. In 10 patients premature partial closure of the valve was observed during ejection. After striking the apex of the cage during early ejection the poppet descended almost half the distance toward the base of the valve and remained in a relatively fixed, partially closed position during the remainder of the ejection period. Instability of the poppets of the Starr-Edwards ball valves has also been observed in some of our patients at the USC-LA County Medical Center.

(c) In Vitro Results

The in vitro pressure drop studies indicate calculated VA's of 1.04 to 2.12 cm^2 for aortic and mitral valves in the 19 to 32 mm size range. As stated by Lefrak and Starr (31) there is no difference in the in vitro pressure drop and regurgitant characteristics of the non-cloth covered (1200/1260, 6120) and the cloth covered (2310/2320, 2400, 6310/20, 6400) prostheses. The in vitro results also indicate low regurgitant volumes (~ 6 cm^3/beat or less), for the Starr-Edwards ball valves. The Starr-Edwards ball valves have no leakage backflow.

There have been a number of flow visualization studies conducted on the Starr-Edwards ball valves in the aortic and mitral positions (40-44). Wieting (44) observed the flow patterns downstream from a 27 mm model 1260 ball valve, under pulsatile flow conditions. During systole he observed a large turbulent wake distal to the ball. He also found that the ball bounced at the apex of the cage and this probably increased size of the turbulent wake. The large amplitude bounces increased the relative velocity between the surface of the ball and the fluid flowing past it. Yoganathan et al., (45,46) and Figliola (47) have also observed the poppet instability phenomena with the model 1260 valve.

As observed by Yoganathan et al., in their studies the instability of the poppet leads to larger pressure drops across the prosthesis. Dellsperger and Wieting (48) studied a model 6400 valve. In the mitral position they observed boundary layer separation resulting in a stagnation point at the apex and a toroidal vortex downstream from the valve during most of diastole. Smeloff et al., (40) under pulsatile flow observed an area of stasis at the apex of the cage and a region of flow separation adjacent to the sewing ring. Wright and Temple studied flow patterns around a 24 mm aortic (model 2400) and a 32 mm mitral (model 6400) valves under pulsatile flow conditions. In the aortic position they observed a small disturbance extending about half the ball diameter immediately downstream from the apex of the cage. This region of flow gradually extended throughout systole until after 250 ms (5/6 of the way through systole) it was about 1.5 ball diameters in length. In the mitral position they observed an annular vortex (caused by flow separation) in the ventricle so that flow occurred retrogradely towards the rear of the cage and poppet. Flow in the annular region between the flow chamber wall and the poppet surface was jet like.

Tillmann (49) has measured the "wall" (i.e. surface) shear stress along the inside of the orifice during systole, using hot-film shear probes. He measured a maximum average shear stress of 850 dynes/cm^2 and a peak shear stress of 1800 dynes/cm^2. The maximum values occurred at peak systole. In a recent study Phillips et al., made velocity measurements downstream from a 27 mm model (1260 valve) under pulsatile flow conditions. Measurements were made 25 mm (about 5 mm downstream from the cage apex), and 30 mm downstream from the valve. They observed a large turbulent wake in this region. Peak velocities of about 350 cm/s were measured near the walls of the flow channel at peak systole (peak flow of about 45 l/min). The flow near the walls was jet like. RMS axial velocities on the order of 125 cm/s were also measured. Average turbulent shear stresses during peak flow were estimated to be on the order of 3000 dynes/cm^2. It is expected that larger turbulent shear stresses would be observed closer to the valve.

Figliola has measured velocity and shear stresses downstream from a 25 mm (model 1260) aortic valve at a steady flow rate of 25 l/min (47). He observed regions of separated flow in the sinus region attached to the sewing ring, along the cage struts, and downstream from the poppet. Maximum wall shear stresses on the order of 500 to 850 dynes/cm^2 were measured. Turbulence intensities as high as 40% and bulk turbulent shear stresses of about 600 dynes/cm^2 (maximum value) were measured 22 mm downstream (about 4 mm downstream from cage apex) from the valve. He also was able to measure a maximum occluder wall shear stress of 3210 dynes/cm^2. Figliola also made velocity and shear measurements downstream of a model 2320 valve (25 mm valve size) at a steady flow rate of 25 l/min. The velocity measurements revealed regions of separated flow in the sinus attached to the sewing ring, distal to the ball, and along the cage struts, similar to those observed with the model 1260 valve. The maximum wall shear stress measured was on the order of 1300 dynes/cm^2. Turbulence intensities as high as 40% and turbulence shear stresses as large as 711 dynes/cm^2 were measured 22.5 mm downstream from the valve. Occluder wall shear stresses were on the order of 2300 dynes/cm^2. Figliola states that the smaller values of wall shear measured with the model 1260 valve as opposed to the model 2320 valve can be attributed to the shorter profile of the model 1260 valve (47). The shorter profile enables the entire occluder to be positioned within the sinus region. Therefore, the blockage due to the occluder is less as the cross-sectional area is larger within the sinus region.

Yoganathan et al., have also made velocity and shear stress measurements downstream from a 27 mm (model 1260) valve in an aortic chamber under steady flow conditions (45,46). Experiments were conducted at steady flow rates of 10 and 25 l/min. They have identified a region of stasis at the apex of the cage, and a region of flow separation which was attached to the aortic side of the sewing ring and the base of the three struts and extended about 2 to 5 mm downstream from the valve along the walls of the flow chamber. At a flow rate of 25 l/min the region of stasis was about 7 to 8 mm in size. Maximum wall shears measured were on the order of 1750 dynes/cm^2, and poppet wall shears were on the order of 2500 to 2800 dynes/cm^2. Turbulence intensity levels as high as 50% were measured in the wake region immediately downstream from the poppet, and in the annular region between the poppet surface. Maximum turbulent shear stresses on the order of 2000 to 5000 dynes/cm^2 (peak values) were measured in these regions.

(d) Correlation

The in vivo and in vitro pressure measurements indicate that like other ball valves, due to its centrally occluding design, the Starr-Edwards ball valves are moderately stenotic in the medium to larger sizes. In the smaller sizes the valves are very stenotic. Patients with this prosthesis would not be able to lead very strenuous life styles. The prosthesis does have low regurgitant volumes, the lowest among mechanical prostheses in current clinical use. The in vivo and in vitro data seem to indicate that the instability of the silicone rubber poppet (1200/1260, 6120) could lead to larger pressure drops across the prosthesis.

The large wall shear stresses created by the Starr-Edwards ball valves could cause lethal damage to the endothelial lining of the vessel wall adjacent to the valve, especially in the aortic position. The bulk turbulent shear stresses are large enough to cause sublethal and/or lethal damage to the red cells and platelets. Damage to the red cells and platelets will reduce their half-lifes, as well as cause hemolysis and thromboembolic complications. The shear stresses immediately adjacent to the valve cage (in the annular region) are large enough to lethally damage any formed elements of blood which may adhere to the valve cage or poppet. The clinical data (17,18-25) indicate very clearly that the cloth covered models (2300-10-20, 2400, 6300-10-20, 6400) create more hemolysis than the non-cloth covered models (1200/1260, 6120). The most probable and logical explanation for this clinical observation is that the porous cloth covering, which is rough, provides an ideal foreign surface for the adhesion of the red cells as they flow past the valve struts. Once adhered, the red cells undergo shear stresses on the order of 10^2-10^3 dynes/cm^2 which lead to their destruction and cause hemolysis.

The regions of stasis at the cage apex and flow separation immediately downstream from the ball could lead to thrombus formation at the apex. The region of flow separation at the base of the three struts and along them could encourage thrombotic material to form at the base and then grow along the struts. The

region of separation attached to the downstream side of the
sewing ring could lead to the excess growth of fibrous tissue
on that portion of the sewing ring. In addition, the flow
separation along the struts of the completely cloth covered strut
valves (2300-10-20, 6300-10-20) could encourage the growth of
excess tissue, especially along the inner aspects, since the
flow and shear are low in those locations. The fibrous tissue
overgrowth problem observed with the completely fabric covered
strut prostheses has mainly occurred on the inner aspects of
the cage. The cloth covering along the inside of the orifice
probably also causes flow separation, and if so could lead to
excess tissue growth along the fabric in the orifice and cause
the valve to become stenotic, as observed clinically.

(2) Kay-Shiley Disc Valve
(a) Valve Description
The first Kay-Shiley Mitral valve was implanted in 1965 and
underwent design and material changes until the final muscle guard
series in 1969. The first (series K) valve consisted of a
Silicone disc held in a Stellite metal cage. The amount of
cloth covering was later increased in an attempt to decrease the
potential for thromboembolism (series T). The major design
change made thereafter was development of the muscle guard to
prevent infringement of the ventricular muscle on the valve. The
muscle guard series MG and TG (MG = Mitral Guards and TG =
Tricuspid Guards) were introduced in 1968 and the extent of cloth
covering was increased in 1969 (MGC, TGC). The last modification
was changing the disc from Silicone to Delrin (MGCD, TGCD).
(b) In Vivo Results
The Kay-Shiley mitral valve had calculated VA's of 0.9 to 2.1 cm^2
in the 28 to 33 mm size range. These results indicate this
prosthesis is more stenotic than the caged ball type valves. Our
study indicates there are very few articles on hemolysis with
the Kay-Shiley valve. The valve did not seem to cause clinically
significant hemolysis, but probably caused mild hemolysis. One
of the major problems with this prosthesis was, however, thromboembolic complications. TEC rates as high as 34.4% per pt. yr.
have been observed with this prosthesis (52). Thrombus formation on the valve superstructure causing dysfunctions of the
Kay-Shiley valve is well documented in the literature
(1,19,35,51-55,57). Thrombi were mainly located at the junction
of the cage struts with the metal orifice ring, up the vertical
struts for variable distances, and occasionally completely
covering the entire metal superstructure. Clots have also been
observed on the disc and on the sewing ring. The prosthesis
has occasionally been completely occluded by thrombotic material.

Excess tissue growth on the sewing ring has also been a
problem with this prosthesis (38,55-58). In some cases the
movement of the disc was severely restricted because of tissue
overgrowth between the disc and sewing ring. In other cases

part of the disc has been trapped by tissue overgrowth and thrombus formation. Such entrapment has transformed the disc into a hinged mechanism, thereby reducing the flow orifice, as well as leading to accelerated edge wear of the disc by the metal struts (31). Excess tissue growth along the sewing ring have on occasions impaired the rotation of the disc. This impairment has led to grooving of the downstream face of the disc from mechanical contact with the horizontal struts (31,38,57).

(c) In Vitro Results

Very few in vitro studies exist on the Kay-Shiley valve. The limited in vitro pressure drop studies indicate VA's of about 1.90 cm^2 for the size 31 mm valves in the mitral position. Weiting has observed the flow patterns around a 28 mm Kay-Shiley valve in an aortic chamber (44). He observed a symmetrical toroidal vortex and a wake downstream from the disc caused by boundary layer separation during systole. He also observed an area of stasis at the center of the distal surface of the disc. The flow was jet like in the regions between the disc and the flow channel walls. Similar flow visualization studies and observations have been made by Duff (59). Figliola (47) has made velocity and shear stress measurements downstream from a 27 mm Kay-Shiley valve (T series) in an aortic chamber under steady flow conditions. He observed a jet type flow between the poppet and flow chamber wall. He also observed flow separation at the sewing ring, and at the junction of the vertical struts and the orifice ring. A large wake with recirculating flow was monitored downstream from the face of the disc. At a flow rate of 25 l/min he measured a maximum wall shear stress of 2548 dynes/cm^2, turbulence intensities of 48% and Reynolds shear stresses of 800 dynes/cm^2. He also was able to measure shear stress of about 775 dynes/cm^2 at the occluder wall surface. The Reynolds stress was measured about 25 mm downstream from the valve. Figliola states that even larger values of Reynolds shear stress could occur closer to the valve occluder. Yoganathan et al., (45,60,61) conducted velocity measurements downstream of a 26 mm Starr-Edwards disc valve in an aortic chamber. The Starr-Edwards disc valve is quite similar to the Kay-Shiley valve. A large region of flow stagnation 20 mm wide was observed across the face of the disc. At a flow rate of 25 l/min a maximum wall shear stress of 3200 dynes/cm^2, and turbulent intensities of 50% were measured. Turbulent shear stresses on the order of 2000 to 5000 dynes/cm^2 were estimated. Pressure drop measurements (45) across this valve indicated it was the most stenotic mechanical valve design (i.e.: disc type valve).

(d) Correlation

The limited in vivo and the very limited in vitro pressure drop results available for the Kay-Shiley disc valve indicate that it is more stenotic than the ball type valves. As stated by

Roberts (1) the disc type valves are the least desirable prosthetic cardiac valves now in use. They are also the most obstructive. The wall shear stresses created by this type of valve could easily damage the endothelial lining of the vessel walls adjacent to the prosthesis. The turbulent shear stresses could cause sublethal and/or lethal damage to red cells and platelets. Such blood element damage could clinically cause hemolytic and thromboembolic problems. The region of stasis across the face of the disc could encourage thrombotic material to form there as has been observed with recovered valves. The regions of flow separation at the junctions of the vertical struts and orifice ring and near the sewing ring could lead to thrombus formation and excess tissue overgrowth at these locations. As stated previously, clinical pathologic findings indicate that these regions are the most prone to thrombus formation and tissue overgrowth with this valve. In addition, Roberts (1,62) states that intimal proliferation of the vessel wall adjacent to valve (mainly in the aortic position) is probably most severe with the disc type valves. The intimal proliferation is caused by large wall shear stresses.

(3) Beall Disc Valve
(a) Valve Description
The low-profile Beall Teflon-disc mitral valve prosthesis was introduced for clinical use in 1967 (model 103). The disc was made of compressed Teflon and the titanium cage was covered with Teflon tubing. The valve ring was totally covered with Dacron velour in an attempt to achieve a low incidence of thromboembolism. In 1968 because of Teflon wear, the thickness and compression of the Teflon disc was increased as was the thickness of the Teflon coating of the titanium cage. Later improvements of the valve design (model 104) were directed toward increasing its frustrum area without chaning its mounting diameter, and on making the materials more durable. The model 105 Beall valve was introduced in 1971. In the model 105 the disc and struts were covered with pyrolitic carbon. After problems of strut fractures were reported, the struts were made stronger and a new method of packaging was begun. The model 106 valve with the thicker more durable struts has been available since 1974 for atrioventricular valve replacement.
(b) In Vivo Results
The clinical pressure drop results obtained with the Beall valve indicate that it is even more stenotic than the Kay-Shiley disc valve. Calculated VA's varied between 1.4 and 2.3 cm^2 for valve sizes in the 31 to 41 mm range. One of the major clinical problems with the Beall disc valve was the excessive amount of hemolysis it caused (63,64,65,66,67). It has been suggested that the Dacron velour cloth covering used was the reason for the excessive hemolysis observed with this valve (31). It has

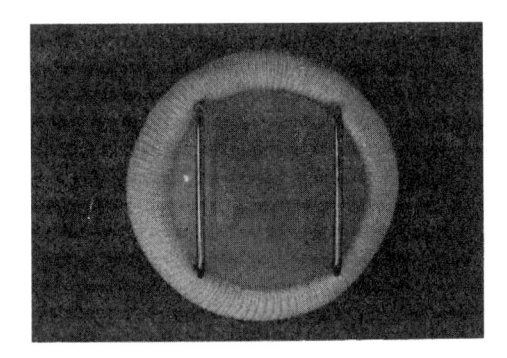

Figure 2. Kay-Shiley disc valve

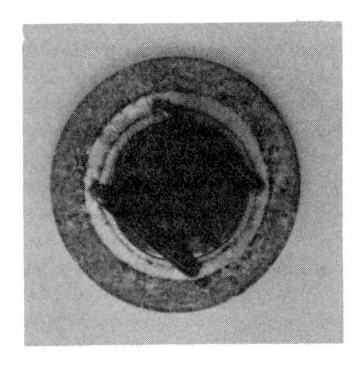

Figure 3. Beall disc valve, model 106

also been suggested that disc wear of the Teflon disc models exacerbated the native hemolysis of this prosthesis (63). Nearly all patients who had this valve suffered at least mild intravascular hemolysis. A comparison of the TEC data tend to indicate that with anticoagulation therapy, thromboembolic complications with the Beall valve were not as severe as those observed with the Kay-Shiley valve. But as stated by Lefrak and Starr (412), only a few publications have appeared in which time-related analysis has been utilized to analyze the rate of postoperative thromboemboli. Thrombus formation causing valve dysfunction has also been documented (53,63,67-70). As stated by Roberts et al., (62) disc type prostheses will develop thrombotic material at the junctions of the vertical struts and the orifice ring, along the vertical struts and across the face of the disc. Usually the amount of thrombus on the struts or primary orifice is not sufficient to interfere with the proper movement of the disc, and clinical evidence of systemic embolic incidents are infrequent when the prosthetic thrombi are small. Large thrombi may, however, obstruct flow through the prosthesis and may immobilize the disc. They also state that prostheses of the disc type may be tilted in the cage by throbmus on one side, or thrombus may fill the entire space between the disc and the ring, causing complete immobility of the poppet (62). As observed with the Kay-Shiley valve, thrombus formation and excess tissue overgrowth may cause improper motion of the disc (proper motion requiring movement up and down the cage, and rotation), thereby leading to grooving and notching of the disc (66,71,72).

(c) In Vitro Results

In vitro fluid dynamic studies on the Beall disc valve are virtually nonexistent in the open literature. It is doubtful if any such tests were even performed by the valve manufacturer when the valves were released in the mid to late 1960's. It is, however, our opinion that the velocity and shear fields downstream from this valve are similar to those observed with the Kay-Shiley and Starr-Edwards disc valves.

(d) Correlation

The Beall disc valve is a very stenotic valve design. If the assumptions about its in vitro fluid dynamic characteristics are correct, the wall and turbulent shear stress created by this valve could easily damage the endothelial lining of the vessel walls, and cause sublethal and/or lethal damage to blood elements, respectively. In addition, if the red cells were to attach themselves to the Dacron velour cloth covering, the shear stresses adjacent to the valve superstructure would be more than sufficient to cause lethal red cell damage (hemolysis). This has been observed clinically with this prosthesis and the cloth covered Starr-Edwards ball valves. The region of flow stasis adjacent to the downstream face of the disc and the regions of flow separation at the junctions of the vertical struts and the orifice ring could lead to a buildup of thrombotic material and excess tissue overgrowth at those locations as has been observed on some recovered Beall valves. The early model Beall valve was briefly utilized in the aortic position but its use in this location was abandoned because of obstructive, thrombogenic and wear characteristics (1,62). Furthermore, Roberts in his pathologic studies observed that disc valves in the aortic position cause intimal proliferation of the aortic root, as a result of excessive wall shear stresses (1,62).

(4) Bjork-Shiley Tilting Disc Valve
(a) Valve Description
The Bjork-Shiley tilting disc prosthesis has been in clinical use since January 1969. The prosthesis has undergone various modifications in design and materials since its initial use. The original Bjork-Shiley valve had a Delrin disc. Although Delrin had excellent wear characterisitcs it had a propensity to absorb moisture during steam autoclaving, a procedure not recommended by the manufacturer. Thus, the disc if improperly sterilized by this method could enlarge and produce temporary irregular valve function. Since the spring of 1971 the disc has been made of pyrolytic carbon which is extremely durable and does not absorb moisture during steam autoclaving. In this valve design a free-floating disc is suspended between two eccentrically situated Stellite struts. The valve presently tilts open to an angle of $60°$ in both aortic and mitral models although in the earlier Delrin disc model the mitral prosthesis was designed to tilt open to an angle of only $50°$. The disc sits inside the base ring in the closed position thus preventing over lapping and reducing mechanical hemolysis. The Stellite base ring is partially covered by a thin Teflon suture ring. This valve design has the advantage of a large ratio of orifice diameter to annulus diameter. When the Bjork-Shiley valve is sutured in place the cage can be rotated within the sewing ring by means of a valve holder in order to ensure free movement of the disc.

In June 1976 Professor Viking O. Bjork implanted the first modified Bjork-Shiley valve with a convexo-concave (C.C.) disc. The modified valve was designed according to Dr. Bjork to improve the conventional Bjork-Shiley valve in three respects: (1) provide increased strength of the valve by making the inlet strut an integral part of the orifice ring and doubling its cross-sectional area (2) improve the hydrodynamics (3) reduction in the area of low flow and stagnation behind the disc. The design change includes the convexo-concave configuration of the disc and a pivot point which has been moved several millimeters downstream so that the disc in the open position is moved further out of the orifice ring. Valves manufactured after September 1975 have a radio-opaque tantalum loop incorporated in the pyrolytic carbon disc to allow evaluation of the opening angle of the disc.

(b) __In Vivo__ Results
Clinical hemodynamic results indicate that the Bjork-Shiley valve has improved pressure drop characterisitcs compared to the centrally occluding (ball and disc) and porcine valve prostheses. Calculated valve areas (VA's) varied from 1.06 to 2.56 cm^2 for aortic valve sizes of 19 to 31 mm, and 1.8 to 2.6 cm^2 for mitral valve sizes of 27 and 29 mm. The limited hemodynamic data tend to indicate no significant differences in the pressure drop characteristics of the spherical and convexo-concave disc aortic valves. Due to its world wide popularity there is a large amount of literature in the medical field on this prosthesis. Hemolysis data indicate that the Bjork-Shiley prosthesis can cause mild to moderate hemolysis. Patients with this prosthesis, however, rarely develop anemia because the body usually compensates adequately for the hemolysis caused by the valve. The prosthesis has a TEC rate of about 4 to 6% per pt. yr. The major problem with the Bjork-Shiley valve is its potential to thrombose, sometimes catastrophically, especially in patients not on anticoagulation therapy (53,55,73-83).

In addition to thrombus formation, excess tissue overgrowth has also been observed on recovered Bjork-Shiley valves. Please note that the above references all pertain to the standard (i.e.: spherical disc) Bjork-Shiley model (except ref. 73,83). There have been no long term studies on the convexo-concave model, and thrombus formation on this model has so far only been reported in two articles (73,83). Thrombus formation mainly occurs on the outflow face of the disc especially in the well, and along the struts in the minor outflow region. However, thrombus formation on both the inflow and outflow faces of the disc has been observed in some recovered valves. Excess tissue overgrowth is observed mainly along the sewing ring of the minor outflow region. The amounts of thrombus formation and/or tissue overgrowth observed on recovered Bjork-Shiley aortic and mitral valves has varied from total valve occlusion to a thin layer. In some instances the combination of thrombus formation and tissue overgrowth has grown in such a manner to impede the complete opening of the tilting disc. In other instances, the disc has been found to be held immobilized in an open position by the vegetation. Therefore, it is of utmost importance that the physician be able to monitor the motion of the disc using cinefluoroscopy.

(c) __In Vitro__ Results
The __in vitro__ pressure drop rsults indicate that the Bjork-Shiley valves have calculated VA's of 1.37 to 3.40 cm^2 for aortic and mitral valves in the 21 to 31 mm size range. There does not seem to be any significant difference in the pressure drop and regurgitation characteristics between the spherical and convexo-concave disc valves. Regurgitation data tend to indicate that

at low heart rates and low cardiac outputs the Bjork-Shiley valve does have a significant regurgitant volume (16). For example, the recent study by Dellsperger et al. showed that the 27 mm Bjork-Shiley (c-c) aortic valve had a regurgitant volume as high as 13.0 cm^3/beat at a heart rate of 50 beats/min (16).

There have been many flow visualization studies conducted on the Bjork-Shiley valve in both the aortic and mitral positions (41,42,48,84-87). Wright has studied the valve (size 25 mm) under pulsatile flow in a curved aorta (41,87). When the valve was oriented so that the disc opened towards the outer curve of the aorta, a clockwise rotating vortex was formed in the ascending aorta during most of systole. Orientation of the disc towards the inside curve produced a relatively narrow, tangential jet. When the valve was mounted to open towards the non-coronary sinus, a double helix swirling flow stream was produced. In the mitral position (size 29 mm valve) he observed that a large two dimensional vortex formed which dominated the left ventricle for most of diastole. Dellsperger and Wieting studied a 29 mm valve in the mitral position (48). They observed a region of stasis underneath the outflow face of the disc during a major portion of diastole. A similar region of stagnation can be observed in the results obtained by Olin in an aortic flow chamber (42). Flow visualization studies under pulsatile flow conditions in our laboratory have shown that there is a large region of stasis underneath the outflow faces of the aortic and mitral discs during the major portions of systole and diastole, respectively (88). The studies have also shown qualitatively that regions of stagnation observed with the convexo-concave valves are smaller than those observed with the sperical disc valves. Schramm et al., studied a 25 mm spherical disc valve in an aortic chamber at a steady flow rate of 18 l/min (85). They have observed jet type flow immediately downstream from the major orifice, which is directed tangentially towards the wall. They have also observed a large region of stagnation across the outflow face of the disc. Measurements on a 25 mm convexo-concave valve under the same conditions showed: (i) a more pronounced jet through the major orifice and (ii) a smaller region of stagnation across the outflow face of the disc.

Figliola has made steady flow velocity and shear stress measurements downstream from a 25 mm spherical disc aortic valve (47,89). At a flow rate of 25 l/min he measured a maximum wall shear stress of 722 dynes/cm^2 and an occluder wall shear stress (resolved on the upper side of occluder) of 440 dynes/cm^2. He also monitored a maximum turbulent shear stress of 545 dynes/cm^2, a 25 mm downstream from the valve. His velocity measurements also showed a large region of stagnation across the outflow face of the disc. Tillman has measured the "wall" (i.e.: surface) shear stresses along the orifice ring in the major and minor outflow regions of an aortic valve under pulsatile flow

(49,90). During systole he measured maximum surface shear stresses of 150 dynes/cm^2 and 50 dynes/cm^2 in the major and minor orifices, respectively. During diastole he measured a maximum shear stress of about 250 dynes/cm^2 in the minor orifice.

Phillips and his co-workers (86,91) made velocity measurements under pulsatile flow conditions downstream from a 25 mm convexo-concave aortic valve. At peak systole (peak flow of 45 l/min) they observed jetting through the major orifice with velocities on the order of 350 cm/s, 14 mm downstream from the valve. RMS measurements of the axial velocity showed large turbulence fluctuations (on the order of 140 cm/s). They estimated the maximum turbulent shear stress during systole to be on the order of 2000 to 6500 dynes/cm^2.

Yoganathan et al., have measured velocities and shear stresses downstream from a 27 mm spherical disc valve as well as a convexo-concave valve in the aortic position. Experiments were conducted at a steady flow rate of 25 l/min, (60,81,92). The measurements with the spherical disc valve identified a zone of stagnation about 20 mm wide near the aortic face of the disc. The average velocities in the major and minor outflow regions were around 100 and 25 cm/s, respectively, and the corresponding peak shear stresses adjacent to the sewing ring were approximately 700 and 150 dynes/cm^2. A maximum wall shear stress of 1390 dynes/cm^2 was measured. With the convexo-concave valve the region of stagnation was observed to be 10 mm wide, and the average velocities in the major and minor outflow regions were around 90 and 40 cm/sec, respectively. Peak shear stresses on surfaces adjacent to the sewing ring in the major and minor outflow regions were about 500-600 and 300-350 dynes/cm^2, respectively. The convexo-concave valve does, however, direct relatively high flow from the major outflow region towards one of the sinuses of Valsalva depending on its orientation. Wall shear stresses on the order of 1750 dynes/cm^2 were observed on the sinus wall towards which the high flow was directed. Turbulent measurements with both models indicated turbulent shear stresses on the order of 500 to 2000 dynes/cm^2 immediately downstream (3 to 15 mm) from the valve.

(d) Correlation

The in vivo and in vitro pressure measurements indicate that in the larger sizes and under resting conditions the pressure drop characteristics of the Bjork-Shiley valve are quite satisfactory. However, under exercise conditions and/or in the smaller sizes the valve could become mild to moderately stenotic. This is especially true in the mitral position. The in vitro study by Dellsperger et al., (16) suggest that at low heart rates and low cardiac outputs the in vivo regurgitation volumes with this prosthesis could become significant. The wall shear stresses created by this valve could cause sublethal and/or lethal damage to the endothelial lining of vessel walls especially in the aortic position. Turbulent shear stresses are large enough to cause sublethal and/or lethal damage to red cells and platelets thereby reducing their half-lifes. Therefore, it is not surprising to observe clinically, hemolysis and thromboembolic problems with this prosthesis.

The in vitro studies have documented conclusively that the Bjork-Shiley valve creates two unequal regions of flow. There is a region of stasis underneath the outflow face of the disc and low flow through the minor outflow region. It is therefore fairly obvious that thrombus formation will occur on the outflow face of the disc and along the struts in the minor outflow region. As observed by Yoganathan et al., once the thrombus formation and tissue overgrowth begins on the downstream side of the valve the flow field becomes even more favorable for further thrombus formation and tissue overgrowth on the valve superstructure (81). The recovered Bjork-Shiley valves which have thrombus on both the outflow and inflow faces of the disc, probably had thrombus occur on the outflow face of the disc first. The initial thrombus formation probably causes unfavorable flow conditions immediately adjacent to the inflow face, thereby causing thrombus formation at that location as well. The low flow and low shear in the minor outflow region would encourage the growth of excess fibrous tissue along the sewing ring in that region. As has been observed in the recovered valves, the combination of thrombus formation and tissue overgrowth can produce catastrophic results.

The smaller region of stagnation, and the better distribution of flow between the major and minor orifices observed with the convexo-concave valve, may hopefully reduce the problems of thrombus formation on the outflow face of the disc, and excess tissue growth along the sewing ring of the minor orifice region.

(5) Hancock Porcine Valve
(a) Valve Description
The Hancock procine bioprosthesis, prepared by the Stabilized Glutaraldehyde Process ("SGP") has been in clinical use since 1970. Porcine valves preserved by the "SGP" process are sutured to a Dacron cloth-covered flexible polypropylene stent. It should be noted that the porcine valve leaflets are composed of natural polymeric materials. A radio-opaque Stellite metal ring encircles the stent and helps maintain orifice shape and proper leaflet coaptation. Model 242 is used for aortic valve replacement while model 342 is used in the mitral and tricuspid valve areas. These models differ only in the shape of their sewing rings. The Hancock Modified Orifice aortic bioprosthesis (HMO-250) differs from the other two models by having replaced the right coronary leaflet, and contains a portion of septal endocardium with a non-coronary leaflet of an appropriate size. This valve modification was accomplished in an attempt to

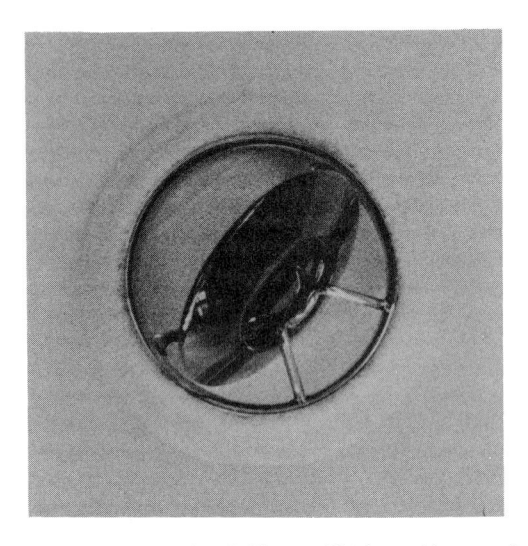

Figure 4. Bjork-Shiley tilting disc valve

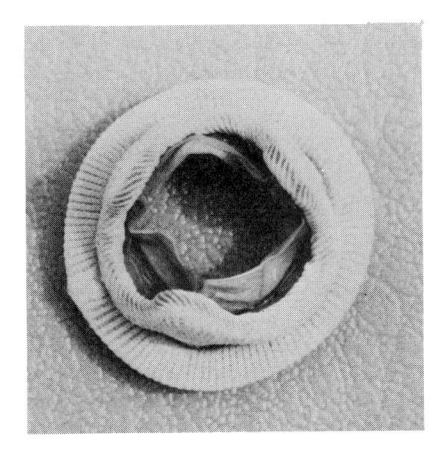

Figure 5. Hancock porcine tissue valve

increase the effective flow orifice for use in patients with a
small aortic annulus. The first clinical implant of a HMO-250
bioprosthesis was in October 1976.
(b) In Vivo Results
Since the Hancock valve is the grandfather of the tissue valve
bioprostheses, there are many articles in the open literature
on its long-term clinical performance. This valve is utilized
in two designs, the standard model and the modified. The
standard model aortic valve has calculated VA's of 0.97 to
1.8 cm^2 for valve sizes of 19 to 27 mm. In the mitral position
calculated VA's ranged from 1.3 to 2.9 cm^2 for valves size
of 23 to 35 mm. The modified orifice aortic valve had VA's
of 0.89 to 1.75 cm^2 for valve sizes of 19 to 25 mm. From a
comparison of the in vivo pressure drop results, it is not
immediately obvious that the modified orifice valves are less
stenotic than the standard model valves. As stated by Rossiter
et al., (93) the hemodynamic differences between the two valve
types are small, and the putative clinical advantages inherent in
the use of the modified orifice valve remain to be completely
defined. Both designs of Hancock valves are, however, more
stenotic compared to the Ionescu-Shiley pericardial valve.
Clinically significant hemolysis is not a major problem with
this valve. Mild amounts of hemolysis have, however, been
documented (94,95). Thromboembolic complications and thrombus
formation on the valve leaflets have also been well documented
(93,96-100). The literature indicates that patients with
Hancock valves have TEC rates of about 2 to 5% per pt. yr.,
the higher rates occurring in mitral valve patients with atrial
fibrillation.

Thrombus formation on the valve structure (i.e., sewing
ring and leaflets) and thrombosis of the Hancock valve, in
both the aortic and mitral position are well documented in the
literature (96,99-107). In a majority of the documented cases
of valve thrombosis, the thrombotic material was found attached
to the downstream sewing ring and up along the outflow surface
of one or more of the leaflets. Thrombotic materials have also
on occasions been observed on the inflow orifice and inflow
surfaces of the leaflets, mainly in the mitral position. On
many occasions the thrombotic material initially started on
the outlfow face of the muscle-shelf leaflets (102,105,108,109).
Thrombus formation on one or more leaflets has at times led
to thrombotic occlusion of the prosthesis and demise of the
patient (102,104-107,109,110). Detailed pathologic studies
on recovered Hancock porcine valves by Ferrans et al.,
(101,103,111), and Spray and Roberts (106) have revealed some
very interesting information. Thrombi are commonly observed
on the outflow surfaces (more so than on the inflow surfaces) of
Hancock porcine valves, in spite of the low incidence of
clinically apparent thromboembolic episodes. Subsequent studies

by others have confirmed these findings (101,104). Ferrans et al., (101) state that their ultra-structural observations point to the possibility that small fibrin deposits and platelet aggregates form continuously on the surfaces of the leaflets and because of the mechanical forces to which they are subjected, the majority of such deposits or aggregates are shed from the surfaces into the blood stream before they have had an opportunity to grow to a larger size. They also state the fact that fibrin thrombi deposits and cells were numerous on the outflow surfaces. This finding is in agreement with the concept that the forces of flow (shear stress) are greater on the inflow than on the outflow surfaces of porcine valves. Therefore fibrin and thrombotic deposits on the outflow surfaces would be less easily removed and would be expected to grow larger and show evidence of organization as observed in their study (101) and the study of Spray and Roberts (106).

One of the major clinical problems of Hancock porcine valves is the calcification of the valve leaflets. The development of calcification appears to be accelerated in children and young adults (96,98,100,103,104,112-115). Ferrans et al.,(103) in an excellent pathologic study observed that the two main sites of deposition of calcium phosphate in porcine valves are in the connective tissue of the cusps and in the small thrombi on the leaflet surfaces. Calcific deposits on the valve leaflets generally lead to prosthetic valve stenosis, because calcification causes impaired leaflet mobility. However, it can also lead to valve regurgitation. Examinations of recovered Hancock valves indicate that calcification is associated with one (generally the muscle-shelf leaflet) or more of the leaflets. It is also not unusual to find that calcification of the leaflets to be associated with thrombotic deposits in and around the same locations. Ferrans et al., (103) observed that calcific deposits associated with vegetation and thrombi, contained remnants of platelets and leukocytes that appeared to have been trapped within a mesh of fibrin standards. Varying degrees of fibrous tissue overgrowth on recovered Hancock porcine valves have also been observed during gross pathologic examinations (97,100,102,104,113,116-119). Although the greatest amount of fibrous tissue overgrowth has been observed around the downstream sewing ring and the outflow bases of the valve cups, tissue overgrowth on the inlet aspect of the sewing ring and valve cusps has also been observed. The fibrous tissue growth may be related to the calcification process (103).

(c) In vitro Results
The standard Hancock valve (model 242 and 342) has VA's in the range of 1.12 to 1.93 cm^2 for both aortic and mitral valves in the 19 and 33 mm size range. The VA's for the modified orifice valves (model 250) varied from 1.02 to 2.01 cm^2 for the 19 to 25 mm valve sizes. Gabbay et al., (120) state that there is no

difference in pressure drop characteristics between the
Carpentier-Edwards and modified orifice Hancock valves of
corresponding sizes. Recent studies in our laboratory have
confirmed these findings. Regurgitation was almost nonexistent
($\sim$ 1 cm^3/beat) for the Hancock valves.

Flow visualization studies (41,85,87,88) indicate that
the flow that emerges from the Hancock valves, standard and
modified orifice, is jet-like. Schramm et al., (85) in their
study showed that there was no reattachment of the jet. At a
steady flow rate of 18l/min they observed a peak jet velocity
of 180 cm/s with a size 25 modified orifice valve. Wright
(41,87) in his studies observed a vortex swirl in addition to
the jet. Yoganathan et al., in their study with a size 27 mm
standard valve and a size 25 mm modified orifice valve, observed
that the jet was not symmetric and was skewed towards one side
(88). Flow separation occurred at the downstream edge of the
leaflets. The annular region between the outflow surface of the
leaflets and the flow channel wall was relatively stagnant. High
speed photography by Rainer et al., (121) showed that there was
high frequency fluttering of the muscle-shelf leaflet during
end-systole in the aortic Hancock valve.

Velocity and shear stress measurements conducted with a
size 27 mm Hancock standard valve in our laboratory give results
similar to those obtained with the Carpentier-Edwards valve (122).
The velocity profiles were jet-like with turbulent shear stresses
on the order of 1000-3000 dynes/cm^2, and wall shear stresses on
the order of 200-600 dynes/cm^2. Flow separation was observed
in the immediate downstream vicinity of the valve, together with
a region of stagnation adjacent to the outflow surfaces of the
leaflets. Leaflet photography studies conducted by Yoganathan
et al., on size 27 and 25 mm Hancock valves showed that the
leaflet opening and closing characteristics leave much to be
desired (88). The leaflets did not open symmetrically or
reproducibly. The leaflet opening areas varied with cardiac
output. In the standard model Hancock valves the muscle-shelf
leaflet was the last open and first to close. The above
observations are similar to those observed with the Carpentier-
Edwards porcine valves.

(d) Correlation

The in vivo and in vitro pressure gradient information clearly
show that the Hancock porcine valves are moderately to highly
stenotic, especially in the smaller sizes. Patients with these
valves will not be able to lead very active lives due to the large
gradients across these valves under exercise conditions. The
stenotic nature of the valve is in part due to the asymmetric
and inadequate opening of the three leaflets. The jet type
flow observed in the flow visualization studies could cause
damage to the aortic or ventricular wall if the jet impinges on
these walls. As stated previously the velocity and shear fields

downstream from the Hancock valves are quite similar to those observed with Carpentier-Edwards valves (88,122). Therefore, sublethal and/or lethal damage could occur to the endothelial lining of the vessel walls, red cells, and platelets, which in turn could lead to hemolytic and thrombotic problems. The observation of platelet aggregates, fibrin thrombi, and remnant platelets on the valve leaflets strongly supports the fact that blood element damage does occur. In addition, the fact that patients with Hancock valves do experience thromboembolic and mild hemolytic problems also strongly suggests that red cells and platelets are being damaged. The region of flow separation which exists adjacent to the downstream sewing ring, could lead to the build up of excess fibrous tissue along the downstream sewing ring and the outflow bases of the cusps. It could also lead to the build up of thrombotic, fibrotic and/or calcific mateiral on the outflow surfaces of the leaflets as observed by Ferrans et al., (101). We would also like to propose that one of the reasons for calcification is the relatively stagnant or low velocity region of flow that exists between the outflow surfaces of the leaflets and the vessel walls. The stiffness of the muscle-shelf leaflet makes its outflow surface a prime location for the deposition of thrombotic material, fibrous tissue growth, and calcium build up.

(6) St. Jude Bi-Leaflet Valve
(a) Valve Description
The St. Jude bi-leaflet valve is a low profile heart valve prosthesis. The valve is made entirely from pyrolytic carbon with a double velour Dacron sewing ring. The leaflets are positioned within the valve housing in such manner as to provide central flow. The leaflets pivot within grooves made in the valve orifice housing. In the fully open position the leaflets are designed to open an angle of 85°. The leaflets are impregnated with tungsten to improve their radio-opacity.

(b) In Vivo Results
The St. Jude prosthesis has been on clinical trials and evaluations since 1977, and was approved for general use in December, 1982. Over 20,000 of these valves have been implanted to date worldwide. The clinical pressure drop results indicate that this valve has probably the best pressure gradient characteristics of any of the prostheses in current clinical use. Calculated VA's in the aortic position have been in the range of 1.5 to 3.6 cm^2, and 2.1 to 4.57 cm^2 in the mitral position for sewing ring sizes of 21 to 27 mm and 23 to 31 mm, respectively. Even under exercise conditions the valve has good pressure drop characteristics. Blood data on patients using this prosthesis indicate that the St. Jude valve creates mild hemolysis in most patients. Thromboembolic data on the valve over the past three years tend to indicate a TEC rate of approximately 1.0 to 2.0% per pt. yr. for patients on

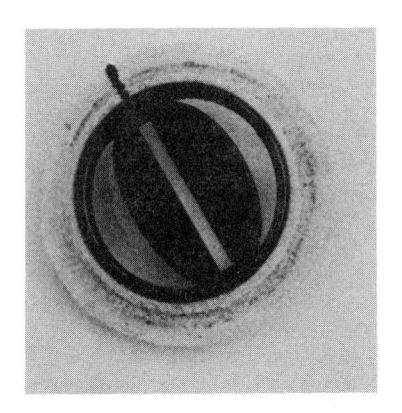

Figure 6. St. Jude bi-leaflet valve

anticoagulation therapy (123-125). Without anticoagulation therapy the valve would probably have an unacceptably high rate of TEC events. Due to the short period of use of this prosthesis no detailed pathological studies on recovered St. Jude valves have been reported in the open literature. Recently there was a case of excess tissue growth on the sewing ring which prevented the opening of one leaflet and allowed the second leaflet to only open about half way (88). The valve was used in the aortic position and was recovered at re-operation.

There have been a few reports in the literature of thrombosis of the St. Jude valve in the aortic, mitral and tricuspid positions (126-128). Nunez et al., reported two cases where one leaflet of the St. Jude valve was jammed by a very small thrombus that fixed the leaflet in a semiclosed position. Both patients were not anticoagulated. Recently, we recovered a St. Jude aortic valve in which both leaflets were jammed in semiopen position due to thrombi in the valve pivot mechanism. Moulton et al., reported a case where the thrombus was adherent at the junction of the two leaflets and which extended 1 cm into the aorta and totaly occluded the right coronary orifice. The patient was on anticoagulation therapy. Ziemer et al., reported a case of intermittent inhibition of leaflet motion due to minimal disproportion between the leaflets and valve ring (129).
(c) In Vitro Results
In vitro flow studies indicate that this valve has the lowest pressure drops of any of the prostheses in current clinical use. Calculated VA's were in the range of 1.4 to 4.45 cm^2 for the size 19 to 31 mm valves, in both aortic and mitral test chambers. A recent study by Dellsperger et al., (16), however, indicates that this valve may have significant regurgitant volumes at low heart rates and low cardiac outputs. For example, at a heart rate of 50 beats/min the size 27 mm St. Jude aortic valve had a total regurgitant volume of 13.2 cm^3/beat.

Flow visualization studies in aortic and mitral chambers under both steady and pulsatile flow indicate smooth central type flow downstream from the valve (48,85,88,130). Initial velocity and shear stress measurements have been made by Yoganathan et al., with size 27 and 25 aortic valves (38,131). The measurements were made under steady flow rates of 10 and 25 l/min. The velocity measurements indicate that the flow field that emerges from the valve is centralized with low turbulence intensities. The measurements showed a region of flow separation immediately downstream from the sewing ring and adjacent to flow channel walls. The region of flow separation is larger adjacent to the center orifice, compared to the separation regions adjacent to the two side orifices. It was also observed that there was more (volumetric) flow through the side orifices compared to the center orifice (approximate ratio of 70:30). Wall shear stresses on the order of 50 to 600 dynes/cm^2 were measured together with estimated turbulent shear stresses of 100-600 dynes/cm^2. Velocity measurements have not been made close to the pivoting mechanism of the valve. Schramm et al., using steady flow conditions, have also observed flow separation occurring from the downstream sewing ring (85). They state that the flow separation generates a ciruclar dead water region which surrounds the main flow. Studies in our laboratory (88) and by Rainer et al., (132) indicate asynchronous closing of the two leaflets in pulsatile flow. We have also observed that particles of dirt in the blood analog fluid cause sticking of the valve leaflets.

(d) Correlation

The *in vivo* and *in vitro* results indicate clearly the superior pressure drop characteristics of the St. Jude prosthesis. This is a tremendous advantage for patients who lead active lives, as well as for children and adults with small valve annuli (123-125). The regurgitation volumes observed *in vitro* at low heart rates could be clinically significant at low cardiac outputs. One of the reasons for this result could be the asynchronous closing of the leaflets. The asynchronous closing of the leaflets is in our opinion an inherent problem with any bileaflet design, since one can not make both leaflets identical. The central flow field created by the valve is an advantage. The wall shears could cause sublethal damage to the endothelial lining of the vessel walls especially in the aortic position, while the turbulent shear stresses could cause sublethal and/or lethal damage to blood elements. It is therefore not surprising to observe mild hemolysis and TEC events, with this prosthesis. The region of flow separation could cause excess tissue growth and/or thrombus formation on the downstream sewing ring which in turn could lead to valve dysfunction by impeding movement of the leaflets. This situation could be aggravated by certain surgical techniques such as using pledgets to sew the valve into place. It is therefore of utmost importance that the physician be able to monitor the movement of the leaflets under cinefluoroscopy. One of the major clinical disadvantages of the St. Jude valve is its poor radiographic visibility, especially if the physician is not familiar with the prosthesis. The problem of sticking leaflets as documented in the medical literature, together with our observations in the pulse duplicator give us concern. A potential failure mode for this prosthesis could be damaged blood elements collecting in the divets (i.e. ears) of the hinge mechanism; forming small thrombi and causing impaired leaflet mobility, as observed by us and other investigators.

Conclusions

Following the collection, analysis, and interpretation of the in vivo and in vitro information and data pertaining to the current state of the art with respect to the safety and performance of prosthetic heart valves (mechanical and tissue), we conclude that:
1. At present we do not have an ideal prosthetic heart valve. During the past 22 years, manufacturers have developed various designs of prosthetic heart valves, some of which perform satisfactorily when implanted surgically in patients suffering from valvular heart disease. Other designs have had to be removed from the open market due to lack of adequate safety and efficacy.
2. There is a lack of in vivo clinical and in vitro fluid dynamic data and information on all designs of prosthetic heart valves in current clinical use. The lack of good quality clinical information and data on some of the older valve types is surprising.
3. Good, long term clinical follow-up data exists only for the following valve types studied: (i) Starr-Edwards ball valves, (ii) Bjork-Shiley tilting disc valve, (iii) Lillehei-Kaster tilting disc valve, and (iv) Hancock porcine valve.
4. There is a lack of good detailed pathologic studies performed on heart valves prostheses recovered at surgery and/or autopsy. The lack of such studies will hinder the progress and development of not only better heart valve prostheses, but also other future artificial devices such as left ventricular assist devices and the total artificial heart.
5. The caliber and quantitative nature of the in vitro fluid dynamic studies has improved a great deal during the past five to six years. There are, however, many pieces of information missing which would give us a better understanding of some of the clinical problems observed with prosthetic heart valves.
6. There seems to be a lack of collaboration between the in vitro investigator and the physician (cardiologist and/or cardiovascular surgeon). Therefore, there are very few articles that attempt to relate specific in vitro flow characteristics to clinical performance and complications. The lack of such information will impede the progress of prosthetic heart valves and similar cardiovascular devices.
7. The available in vivo hemodynamic and in vitro pressure drop results from all valves when analyzed in a combined overall manner indicate that the prostheses studied could be arranged in the following broad categories of decreasing stenoticity (The valves in each category are listed in alphabetical order): (i) caged disc valves (ii) caged

ball valves, Lillehei Kaster tilting disc valve and porcine valves (iii) Bjork-Shiley tilting disc valve and Ionescu-Shiley pericardial valve (iv) Medtronic-Hall tilting disc valve (v) St. Jude bileaflet valve.
8. In terms of regurgitation, in vitro studies indicate that the valves can be arranged in the following broad categories of increasing regurgitation (The valves in each category are listed in alphabetical order): (i) porcine valves (ii) Ionescu-Shiley pericardial valve (iii) Beall disc valve, Braunwald-Cutter ball valve, Kay-Shiley disc valve, and Starr-Edwards ball valve (iv) Bjork-Shiley, Medtronic-Hall, and Lillehei-Kaster tilting disc valves, and the St. Jude bileaflet valve.
9. All prosthetic valves (mechanical and tissue) in current clinical use cause sublethal and/or lethal damage to blood elements such as red cells and platelets. The shear fields created by the valves (10^2-10^3 dynes/cm^2) are all capable of causing such damage. Sublethal damage to red cells could in time lead to mild hemolysis. Similarly, sublethal damage to platelets could over a period of time lead to thromboemboli and TEC's.
10. All peripheral flow type valves cause damage to the endothelial lining of the proximal ascending aorta. This is directly related to the elevated wall shear stresses (10^3 dynes/cm^2) in the immediate downstream vicinity of these valves. They may also cause sublethal and/or lethal damage to the ventricular wall. Other mechanical valve designs and tissue bioprostheses could cause sublethal and/or lethal damage to the endothelial lining of the aortic wall. The jet type flow from the tissue valves in the aortic and mitral positions could cause damage to the walls of the ascending aorta and left ventricle, respectively. Depending on the orientation of the valve, the flow in the major orifice region of a tilting disc mitral valve could also cause damage to the ventricular wall.
11. All prosthetic valves in current clinical use cause hemolysis and TEC's, and are prone to the problems of thrombus formation and excess tissue growth on the valve superstructure.
12. In many cases the hemolysis caused by the prosthesis is mild or moderate, and is generally compensated for quite adequately by natural regeneration in the bone-marrow. Cloth covering on the valve superstructure (such as with the Starr-Edwards and Beall valves) will lead to an increase in hemolysis depending on the structure and surface characteristics of the fabric. Hemolysis, however mild, is not innocuous. It is the forerunner in one of the proposed mechanisms for platelet aggregation and coagulation, which in turn could lead to the formation of thromboemboli.

13. Mechanical valves in current clinical use have TEC rates of about 2 to 8% per pt. yr. for patients on anticoagulation therapy. Tissue valves have TEC rates of about 2 to 5.5% per pt. yr. without the use of long term anticoagulation therapy.
14. Thrombus formation and tissue overgrowth on the valve superstructure are most often found in regions of flow stasis, very low flow and shear, and flow separation.
15. Mechanical damage to the blood elements as well as to the endothelial tissue of the adjacent vessel wall, may in addition trigger complex biochemical reactions which could lead to the excess fibrous tissue overgrowth observed on recovered valves.
16. Tissue valves are prone to calcification, especially in children and young adults. Calcification mainly occurs on the outflow surfaces of the leaflets. Therefore, it is very probable that the relatively stiff nature of the current tissue valve leaflets, together with the region of flow separation and/or flow stagnation which occurs between the outflow surfaces of the leaflets and the vessel wall, could lead to the deposition of calcific, thrombotic and fibrotic material on the outflow surfaces.

Acknowledgments

This study was supported by the Bureau of Medical Devices, FDA (contract #223-81-5000).

Literature Cited

1. Roberts, W. C. Am. J. Cardiol. 1976, 38, 633.
2. Blackshear, P. L. Chemistry of Biosurfaces 1972, 2, 523.
3. Blackshear, P. L. "Mechanical Hemolysis in Flowing Blood"; Fung, Y. C.; Perrone, N.; Anliker, M., Eds.; Biomechanics-Its Foundations and Objectives, Prenctice-Hall: Englewood Cliffs, NJ, 1972; p. 501.
4. Nevaril, G. C.; Hellums, J D.; Alfrey, C. P., Jr.; Lynch, E. C. Am. Inst. Chem. Eng. J. 1969, 15, 707.
5. Hellums, J. D.; Brown, C. H. III. "Blood Cell Damage by Mechanical Forces"; Hwang, N. H. C.; Normann, N. A., Eds.; Cardiovascular Flow Dynamics, University Park Press: Baltimore, MD, 1977; p. 799.
6. Hung, T. C.; Hochmuth, R. M.; Joist, J. H.; Sutera, S. P. Trans. Am. Soc. Int. Organs 1976, 12, 285.
7. Ranstack, J. M.; Zuckerman, L.; Mockros, L. F. J. Biomech. 1979, 12, 113.
8. Mohandas, N.; Hochmuth, R. M.; Spaeth, E. E. J. Biomech. Mat. Res. 1974, 8, 119.
9. Lloyd, J. R.; Mueller, T. J.; Johnson, P. C.; MacDonell, E. H. "Shear Induced Variations in Red Blood Cell Morphology"; Advances in Bioengineering, ASME, 1976, p. 30.
10. McIntyre, L., private communication.
11. Fry, D. L. Circ. Res. 1968, 22, 165.
12. Fry, D. L. Circ. Res. 1969, 24, 93.
13. Woolf, N.; Path, M. C.; Carstairs, K. C. Am. J. Path. 1967, 51, 373.
14. Yoganathan, A. P. "Prosthetic Heart Valves: A Study of In Vitro Performance", Phase I Final Report, FDA Contract #223-81-5000, April 1982 (NTIS #PB 83-134478).
15. Cohen, M. V.; Gorlin, R. Am. Heart J. 1972, 84, 439.
16. Dellsperger, K. C.; Wieting, D. W.; Baehr, D. A.; Bard, R. J.; Brugger, J-P; Harrison, E. C. Am. J. Cardiol. 1983.
17. Santinga, J. T.; Batsakis, J. T.; Flora, J. D.; Kirsh, M. M. Chest 1976, 69, 56.
18. Boncheck, L. I.; Starr, A. Am. J. Cardiol. 1975, 35, 843.
19. Roberts, W. C.; Bulkley, B. H.; Morrow, A. G. Prog. Cardiovasc. Disc. 1973, 15, 539.
20. Crexells, C.; Aerichide, N.; Bonny, Y.; Lepage, G.; Campeau, L. Am. Heart J. 1970, 84, 161.
21. Walsh, J. R., Starr, A.; Ritzmann, L. W. Circulation 1969, 39-40 (Suppl I), I-135.
22. Dale, J.; Myhre, E. Am. Heart J. 1978, 96, 24.
23. Ahmad, R.; Manohitharajah, S. M.; Deverall, P. B.; Watson, D. A. J. Thorac. Cardiovasc. Surg. 1976, 71, 212.

24. Starr, A.; Bonchek, L. I.; Anderson, R. P.; Wood, J. A.; Chapman, R. D. Ann. Thorac. Surg. 1975, 19, 289.
25. Rao, K. M. S.: Learoyd, P. A.; Rao, R. S.; Rajah, S. M.; Watson, D. A. Thorax 1980, 35, 290.
26. Herri, R. H.; Starr, A.; Pierie, W. R.; Wood, J. A.; Bigelow, J. C. Ann. Thorac. Surg. 1968, 6, 199.
27. Isom, O. W.; Spencer. F. C.; Glassman, E.; Teiko, P., Boyd, A. D.; Cunningham, J. N.; Reed, G. E. Ann. Surg. 1979, 186, 310.
28. Starr, A.; Grunkemeier, G.; Lambert, L.; Okies, J. E.; Thomas, D. Circulation 1975, 54 (Suppl III), III-47.
29. Behrendt, D. M.; Austen, W. G. Prog. Cardiovasc. Dis. 1979, 15, 369.
30. Starr, A.; Grunkemier, G. L.; Lambert, L. E.; Thomas, D. R.; Sugimara, S.; Lefrak, E. A. Circulation 1977, 56, (Suppl II), II-133.
31. Lefrak, E. A.; Starr, A. Cardiac Valve Prostheses 1979, Appleton-Century-Crofts, New York.
32. Stein, D. W.; Rahimtoola, S. H.; Kloster, F. E.; Seldon, R.; Starr, A. Surgery 1976, 71, 680.
33. Smithwick, W.; Kouchoukos, N. T.; Karp, R. B.; Pacifico, A. D.; Kirklin, J. W. Ann. Thorac. Surg.1975, 20, 249.
34. Limet, R.; Lepage, G.; Grondin, C. M. Ann. Thorac. Surg. 1977, 23, 529.
35. Roberts, W. C.; Morrow, A. G. Adv. Cardiol. 1972, 7, 226.
36. Roberts, W. C.; Morrow, A. G. Circulation 1967, 48,(Suppl I), I-48.
37. Roberts, W. C.; Morrow, A. G. Johns Hopkins Med. J. 1967, 121, 271.
38. Yoganathan, A. P.; Harrison, E. C. Proc. NBS Conference on Implant Retrieval 1980, p. 175.
39. Hamby, R.; Lee, R. L.; Aintablain, A. Am. J. Cardiol. 1974, 34, 276.
40. Smeloff, E. A.; Huntley, A. C.; Davey, T. B.; Kaufmann, B.; Gerbode, F. J. Thorac. Cardiovasc. Surg. 1966, 52, 841.
41. Wright, J. T. M.; Temple, L. J. Engineering in Med. 1977, 6, 31.
42. Olin, C. Scan. J. Thor. Cardiovasc. Surg. 1971, 5, 1.
43. Duff, W. R.; Fox, R. W. J. Thorac. Cardiovasc. Surg. 1972, 63, 131.
44. Weiting, D. Ph.D. Thesis, University of Texas at Austin, Texas, 1969.
45. Yoganathan, A. P. Ph.D. Thesis, California Institute of Technology, California, 1978.
46. Yoganathan, A. P.; Reamer, H. H.; Corcoran, W. H.; Harrison, E. C.; Shulman, I. A.; Parnassus, W. Artif. Organs 1981, 5, 6.
47. Figliola, R. S. Ph.D. Thesis, University of Notre Dame, Indiana, 1979.

48. Dellsperger, K. C.; Wieting, D. W. Adv. Bio. Eng. 1978, p. 31.
49. Tillmann, W. Proc. 1st Int. Conf. Mechanics in Med. and Biol. 1978, p. 233.
50. Brown, J. W.; Myerowitz, P. D.; Cann, M. S.; Colvin, S. B.; McIntosh, C. L.; Morrow, A. G. Surgery 1974, 76, 983.
51. Bjork, V. O.; Olin, C.; Astrom, H. Scan. J. Thor. Cardiovasc. Surg. 1969, 3, 93.
52. Bowen, T. E.; Zajtchuk, R.; Brott, W. H.; deCastro, C. M. J. Thorac. Cardiovasc. Surg. 1980, 80, 45.
53. Messmer, B. J.; Okies, J. E.; Hallman, G. L.; Cooley, D. A. Ann. Thorac. Surg. 1971, 13, 268.
54. Lee, S. J. K.; Lees, G.; Callaghan, J. C.; Couves, C. M.; Sterns, L. P.; Rossall, R. E. J. Thorac. Cardiovasc. Surg. 1974, 67, 970.
55. Yoganathan, A. P.; Harrison, E. C.; Corcoran, W. H., Ed. Procceedings of a Symposium of the 14th Annual Meeting of the Association for the Advancement of Medical Instrumentation, Prosthetic Heart Valves, 1980.
56. Wukash, D. C.: Sandiford, F. M., Reul, G. J., Jr.; Hallman, G. L., Cooley, D. A. J. Thorac. Cardiovas. Surg. 1975, 69, 107.
57. Edmiston, W. A.; Harrison, E. C.; Batista, E.; Sarma, R.; Kay, J. H.; Lau, F. Y. K. Scan. J. Thor. Cardiovasc. Surg. 1980, 14, 241.
58. Vogel, J. H. K.; Paton, B. C.; Overy, H. R.; Blount, S. G., Jr. Circulation 1969, 39-40, (Suppl I), I-141.
59. Duff, W. R. Ph.D. Thesis, Purdue University, Indiana, 1969.
60. Yoganathan, A. P.; Corcoran, W. H.; Harrison, E. C. J. Bio. Eng. 1978, 2, 369.
61. Yoganathan, A. P.; Corcoran, W. H.; Harrison, E. C. J. Biomech. 1979, 12, 135.
62. Roberts, W. C.; Fishbein, M. C.; Golden, A. Am. J. Cardiol. 1975, 35, 740.
63. Clark, R. E.; Pavlovic, T. A.; Knight, B. E.; Joist, J. H.; Burrows, S. D.; McKnight, R. C.; Brown, E. B. Circulation 1977, 56, (Suppl II), II-140.
64. Henderson, B. J.; Mitha, A. S.; leRoux, B. T.; Gotsman, M. S. Thorax 1973, 28, 488.
65. Williams, J. C., Jr.; Vernon, C. R.; Caicoff, G. R.; Bradley, T. D.; Wheat, M. W., Jr.; Ramsey, H. W. J. Thorac. Cardiovasc. Surg. 1971, 61, 393.
66. Kalmanson, D., ed. The Mitral Valve: A Pluridisciplinary Approach, Publishing Sciences Group, Inc.; Acton, MA, 1976.
67. Rossi, N. P.; Kongtahworn, C.; Ehrenhaft, J. L. J. Thorac. Cardiovasc. Surg. 1974, 67, 83.
68. Fernandez, J.; Morse, D.; Spagna, P.; Lemole, G.; Gooch, A.; Yang, S. S.; Maranhao, V. J. Thorac. Cardiovasc. Surg. 1976, 71, 218.

69. Nichols, H. T.; Fernandez, J.; Morse, D.; Gooch, A. S. Chest 1972, 62, 277.
70. Beall, A. C., Jr.; Morris, G. C., Jr.; Howell, J, F., Jr.; Guinn, G. A.; Noon, G. P.; Reul, G. J., Jr.; Greenberg, J. J.; Ankeney, J. L. Ann. Thorac. Surg. 1979, 15, 601.
71. Silver, M. D.; Wilson, G. J. Circulation 1977, 56, 617.
72. Smiley, W. H.; Gilbert, C. A.; Symbas, P. N. Southern Med. J. 1977, 70, 801.
73. Bjork, V. O.; Henze, A. J. Thorac. Cardiovasc. Surg. 1979, 78, 331.
74. Chandraratna, P. A. N.; Lopez, J. M.; Hildner, F. J.; Samet, P.; Ben-Zvi, J. Am. Heart J. 1976, 91, 318.
75. Shoen, F. J.; Braunwald, N. S. J. Biomed. Mater. Res. 1983, 17, 715.
76. Ben-Zvi, J.; Hildner, F. J.; Chandrarathana, P. A.; Samet, P. Am. J. Cardiol. 1974, 34, 538.
77. Dale, J. Am. Heart J. 1977, 93, 715.
78. Aberg, B.: Henze, A.; Bjork, V. O. San. J. Thor. Cardiovasc. Surg. 1977, 11, 1.
79. Roberts, W. C.; Hammer, W. J. Am. J. Cardiol. 1976, 37, 1024.
80. Moreno-Cabral, R. J.; McNamara, J. J.; Mamiya, R. T.; Brainard, S. C.; Chung, G. T. J. Thorac. Cardiovasc. Surg. 1978, 75, 321.
81. Yoganathan, A. P.; Corcoran, W. H.; Harrison, E. C.; Carl, J. R. Circulation 1978, 58, 70.
82. Karp, R. B.; Cyrus, R. J.; Blackstone, E. H.; Kirklin, J. W.; Kouchoukos, N. T. J. Thorac. Cardiovasc. Surg. 1981, 81, 602.
83. Aberg, B. Scan. J. Thor. Cardiovasc. Surg. Suppl. 1980, 25, 1.
84. Bjork, V. O. J. Thorac. Cardiovasc. Surg. 1970, 60, 335.
85. Schramm, D.; Baldauf, W.; Meisner, H. Thorac. Cardiovasc. Surg. 1980, 28, 133.
86. Alchas, P. G.; Snyder, A. J.; Phillips, W. M. in "Pulsatile Prosthetic Valve Flows: Laser Doppler Studies"; Schneck, D. J., Ed.; Bio Fluid Mecahnics, Pergamon Press: New York, 1980; p. 243.
87. Wright, J. T. M. Trans. Am. Soc. Artif. Intern. Organs. 1977, 23, 89.
88. Yoganathan, A. P., unpublished data.
89. Figliola, R. S., Mueller, T. J. J. Bio. Mech. Eng. 1977, 99, 173.
90. Tillmann, W.; Runge, J.; Reul, H. Proc. ESAO:IV 1977, p. 246.
91. Phillips, W. M.; Snyder, A.; Alchas, P.; Rosenberg, G.; Pierce, W. S. Trans. Am. Soc. Artif. Inter. Organs 1980, 26, 43.
92. Yoganathan, A. P.; Reamer, H. H.; Corcoran, W. H.; Harrison, E. C. Scan. J. Thor. Cardiovasc. Surg. 1980, 14, 1.

93. Rossiter, S. J.; Miller, D. C.; Stinson, E. B.; Oyer, P. E.; Reitz, B. A.; Moreno-Cabral, R. J.; Mace, J. G.; Robert, E. W.; Tsagaris, T. J.; Sutton, R. B.; Alderman, E. L.; Shumway, N. E. J. Thorac. Cardiovasc. Surg. 1980, 80, 54.
94. Magilligan, D. J., Jr.; Fisher, E.; Alam, M. J. Thorac. Cardiovasc. Surg. 1980, 79, 628.
95. Rhodes, G. R., McIntosh, C. L. J. Thorac. Cardiovasc. Surg. 1977, 73, 312.
96. Sade, R. M.; Greene, W. B.; Kurtz, S. M. Am. J. Cardiol. 1979, 44, 761.
97. Stinson, E. B.; Griepp, R. B.; Oyer, P. E.; Shumway, N. E. J. Thorac. Cardiovasc. Surg. 1977, 73, 54.
98. Oyer, P. E.; Stinson, E. B.; Reitz, B. A.; Miller, D. C.; Rossiter, S. J.; Shumway, N. E. J. Thorac. Cardiovasc. Surg. 1979, 78, 343.
99. Duran, C. G.; Pomar, J. L.; Revuelta, J. M.; Gallo, I.; Poveda, J.; Ochoteco, A.; Ubago, J. L. J. Thorac. Cardiovasc. Surg. 1980, 79, 326.
100. Lakier, J. B.; Khaja, F.; Magilligan, D. J., Jr., Goldstein, S. Circulation 1980, 62, 313.
101. Ferrans, V. J.; Spray, T. L.; Billingham, M. E.; Roberts, W. C. Am. J. Cardiol. 1978, 41, 1159.
102. Hetzer, R.; Hill, J. D.; Kerth, W. J.; Wilson, A. J.; Adappa, M. G.; Gerbode, F. Ann. Thorac. Surg. 1978, 2, 317.
103. Ferrans, V. J.; Boyce, S. W.; Billingham, M. E.; Jones, M.; Ishihara, T.; Roberts, W. C. Am. J. Cardiol. 1980, 46, 721.
104. Magilligan, D. J., Jr.; Lewis, J. W., Jr.; Jara, F. M.; Lee, M. W.; Riddle, J. M. Ann. Thorac. Surg. 1980, 30.
105. McComb, R. D.; Stahmann, F. D.; O'Connor, W. N.; Todd, E. P. Ann. Thorac. Surg. 1979, 27, 191.
106. Spray, T. L.; Roberts, W. C. Am. J. Cardiol. 1977, 40, 319.
107. Fishbein, M. C.; Gissen, S. A.; Collins, J. J., Jr.; Barsamian, E. M.; Cohn, L. W. Am. J. Cardiol. 1977, 40, 331.
108. Cohn, L. H.; Koster, J. K.; Mee, R. B. B.; Collins, J. J. Circulation 1979, 60 (Suppl I), I-93.
109. Hetzer, R.; Hill, J. D.; Kerth, W. J.; Ansbro, J.; Adappa, M. G.; Rodvien, R.; Kamm, B.; Gerbode, F. J. Thorac. Cardiovasc. Surg. 1978, 75, 651.
110. Edmiston, W. A.; Harrison, E. C.; Duick, G. F.; Parnassus, W., Lau, F. Y. K. Am. J. Cardiol. 1978, 41, 508.
111. Ferrans, V. J.; Boyce, S. W.; Billingham, M. E.; Spray, T. L.; Roberts, W. C. Am. J. Cardiol. 1979, 43, 1123.
112. Sanders, S. P.; Levy, R. J.; Freed, M. D.; Norwood, W. I.; Castaneda, A.R. Am. J. Cardiol. 1980, 46, 429.
113. Silver, M. M.; Pollock, J.; Silver, M. D.; Williams, W. G.; Trusler, G. A. Am. J. Cardiol. 1980, 46, 429.

114. Thandroyen, F. T.; Whitton, I. N.; Pirie, D.; Rogers, M. A.; Mitha, A. S. Am. J. Cardiol. 1980, 45, 690.
115. Geha, A. S.; Laks, H.; Stansel, H. C., Jr.; Cornhill, J. F.; Kilman, J. W.; Buckley, M. J.; Roberts, W. C. J. Thorac. Cardiovasc. Surg. 1979, 78, 351.
116. Johnson, A. D.; Peterson, K. L.; LeWinter, M.; DiDonna, G. J.; Blair, G.; Niwayama, G. Circulation 1975, 51, (Suppl I), I-40.
117. Johnson, A.; Thompson, S.; Vieweg, W. V. R.; Daily, P., Oury, J.; Peterson, K. J. Thorac. Cardiovasc. Surg. 1978, 75, 599.
118. McIntosh, C. L.; Michaelis, L. L.; Morrow, A. G.; Itscoitz, S. B.; Redwood, D. R.; Epstein, S. E. Surgery 1975, 78, 768.
119. Pipkin, R. D.; Buch, W. S.; Fogarty, T. J. J. Thorac. Cardiovasc. Surg. 1976, 71, 179.
120. Gabbay, S.; McQueen, D. M.; Yellin, E. L.; Frater, R. W. M. Circulation 1979, 60, (Suppl I), I-62.
121. Rainer, W. G.; Christopher, R. A.; Sadler, T. R., Jr.; Hilgenberg, A. D. Ann. Thorac. Surg. 1979, 28, 274.
122. Yoganathan, A. P.; Woo, Y-R.; Williams, F. P.; Stevenson, D. M.; Franch, R. H.; Harrison, E. C. To be published in Artificial Organs 1983.
123. St. Jude Medical, Inc., 1980, International Valve Symposium, March 5-8, 1980, Scottsdale, Arizona.
124. St. Jude Medical, Inc., First European Symposium, June 21, 1980, Paris, France.
125. Chaux, A.; Gray, R. J.; Matloff, J. M.; Feldman, H.; Sustaita, H. J. Thorac. Cardiovas. Surg. 1981, 81, 202.
126. Nunez, L., M.D.; Iglesias, A., M.D.; Sotillo, J., M.D. Ann. Thorac. Surg. 1979, 29, 567.
127. Commerford, P. J., M.B., Ch.B.; Lloyd, E. A., B.M.; De Nobrega, J. A., M.B., Ch.B. Chest, 1981, 80, 326.
128. Moulton, A. L., M.D., Singleton, R. T., M. D., Oster, W. F., M.D. J. Thorac. Cardiovasc. Surg. 1982, 83, 472.
129. Ziemer, G., M.d., Luhmer, I., M.D., Oelert, H., M.D., Borst, H. G., M.D. Ann. Thorac. Surg. 1982, 33, 391.
130. Emery, R. W., Palmquist, W. E., Mettler, E., Nicoloff, D. M. Trans. Am. Soc. Artif. Intern. Organs 1978, 24, 550.
131. Yoganathan, A. P.; Chaux, A.; Gray, R. J.; De Robertis, M.; Matloff, J. M. Artif. Organs 1982, 6, 288.
132. Rainer, W. G. J. Thorac. Cardiovasc. Surg. 1981, 82, 462.

RECEIVED March 19, 1984

Polymeric Membranes for Artificial Lungs

DON N. GRAY

Owens-Illinois, Inc., Corporate Technology, Toledo, OH 43666

Artificial membrane lungs are devices that perfuse circulating blood by membrane transport of gases. The development of membrane lungs was prompted by a need for an efficient device that could be used longer and that would damage the blood less than the direct blood-gas contact oxygenators. The evolution of the membrane lung during the last twenty-five years was dependent on advances made in permselective and microporous polymers with the required characteristics for the critical membrane portion of the device.

In most commercial membrane artificial lungs, the most significant resistant to gas-transfer is the laminar boundary layer of blood near the membrane. Artificial lungs designed to improve the efficiency of gas transfer per unit area of membrane by minimizing the effect of the stagnant blood boundary layer are now available. These new designs take advantage of the inherently high permeability of new membrane materials.

Breathing is something we do continually from birth to death about ten times a minute, 600 times an hour or 14,000 times a day to change the composition of the gaseous mixture in contact with our lungs. The lung is one of the most complex vital organs and the one often assaulted by polluted air, biological enemies and individual self-destructive habits and lack of concern.

Certainly with the modern emphasis on artificial body replacement parts and the success of implanted bits of hardware and assist devices for the heart (valves, heart bypass and pacemakers) and kidneys (renal dialysis), a substitute device for the natural lung should be considered. Artificial lungs are used daily for short-term (3-4 hours) heart-lung bypas in large, specialized health care centers. These are extracorporeal

0097-6156/84/0256-0151$06.00/0
© 1984 American Chemical Society

devices like kidney dialysis units rather than implants like heart assist devices. These devices function like fish "gills" exchanging blood gases directly (Figure 1) rather than assisting respiration like a bellows or respirator. The technology of these devices is now at the state, many experts believe, that artificial kidneys were thirty years ago.[1] The widespread use and acceptance of this technique will depend to a large extent on the availability of simpler, easier to use, safer and lower cost devices.

The primary purpose of the natural lung is to bring air into contact with the lung membrane. Blood on the other side of the membrane releases carbon dioxide and takes up oxygen. Two fluid movement systems are involved in this dynamic process, one moving air and the other (the heart) moving blood. The surface area of the natural lung is very high (over 70 square meters), while the artificial lung membrane surface area is much lower (3-6 square meters).

Fortunately, artificial membrane lungs can function to achieve adequate gas exchange with lower surface areas because, while the natural lung receives inspired air containing only 21% oxygen, the membrane of the artificial lung sees 100% oxygen.

The development of apparatus to oxygenate blood preceded modern advances in cardiac and thoracic surgery and was absolutely necessary for open heart surgery. Between the 1930's and 1950's, surgeons experimented with blood oxygenators by taking the straight forward approach of contacting whole venous blood with air or oxygen and recirculating the oxygenated form into the body's circulatory system. This procedure gave the surgeon what he needed most, time for surgical repair of a still heart. To increase the blood-gas contact surface area in these devices, oxygen was bubbled through the blood (bubble oxygenators)[2] or discs were used to constantly expose the blood surface to the gas phase (disc oxygenators)[3]. Direct contact of blood and gas leads to protein denaturation and blood cell destruction which limits the use of bubble and disc oxygenators to a maximum of six hours; perfectly satisfactory for most surgical procedures.

It is interesting that other approaches were also tried with some success, such as using a human donor to constantly "breathe" for a patient via cross blood circulation [19,20]. Even more daring was successful ex-vivo use of dissected, specially treated animal lungs for blood oxygenation[21], an intellectual precursor in the development of the artificial membrane lung.

As early as 1955, Kolff and Balzer[4] described a device patterned after an early renal dialysis unit (the Inouye artificial kidney) wherein polyethylene tubing was used in a coil configuration. While the concept was sound, the membrane material choices available at that time were limited.

In 1956 Clowes and coworkers[5] described an oxygenator using flat sheets of membrane to separate the blood and gas (Figure 2). Clowes examined Teflon, ethyl cellulose, polyethylene, cello-

9. GRAY *Polymeric Membranes for Artificial Lungs*

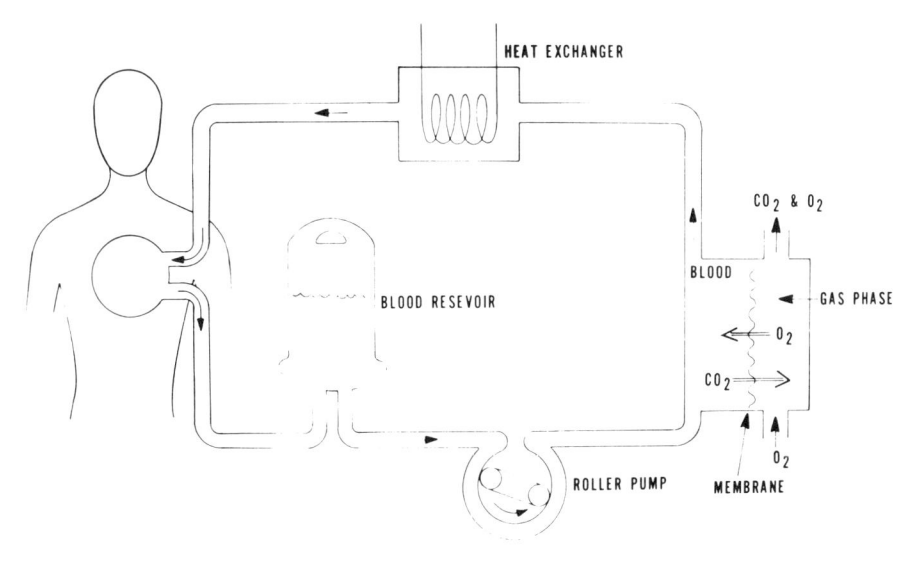

Figure 1. Artificial membrane lung flow diagram.

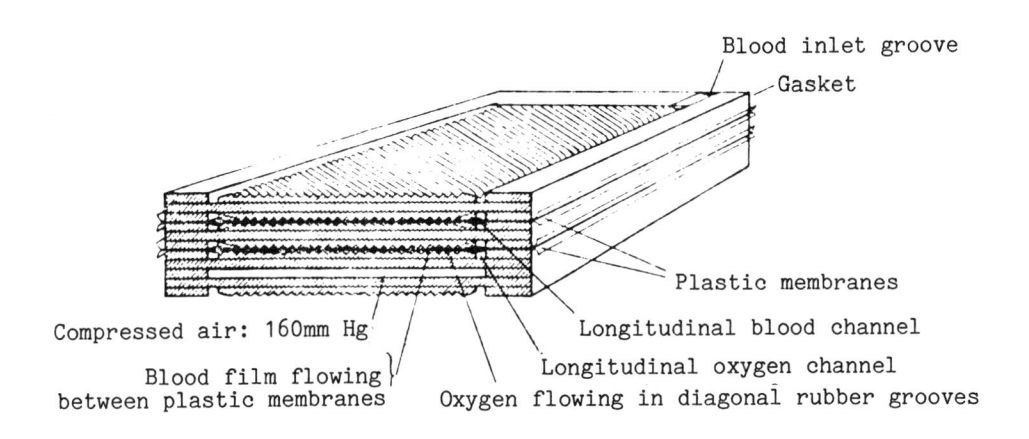

Figure 2. The Clowes membrane oxygenator. (Reproduced with permission from Ref. 5. Copyright 1956, J. Thoracic Surg.)

phane, PVC, polystyrene, Mylar and chlorinated rubber. Note that some of these materials are considered barrier polymers (Mylar and chlorinated rubber). However, ethyl cellulose and Teflon gave promising results. These early workers were using the permselective properties of polymeric membranes for gas, although one might suspect that a portion of the gas passage was due to diffusion via microporous defects in the films. Table 1 is a comparison of the permeability one hundred times that of Teflon .

It is interesting to compare the historical time table for clinical advances versus the commercial status of membrane material at the same point in time. (Table 2 - Significant Milestones - Development of Artificial Membrane Lungs). Note that the first synthetic material used for blood oxygenation (albeit inadvertently) was cellophane, and the mode of oxygen transfer must have been via solubility in the hydrated "aqueous phase" of the swelled polymer. By 1955, the clinicians had experimented with and conceptually optimized the basic geometries of membrane oxygenators. However, the membrane materials available to them were those offered by industry for other purposes, usually packaging. The criteria for choosing the materials were strength, consistent quality (i.e. lack of pin-holes) and thinness. If the materials had some degree of permeability, all the better. The period 1955-1956 was important to the eventual development of superior permselective membranes. Professor Kammermeyer did his first studies on the permeability of silicone films to gases about this time[6] and published his much referenced article "Silicone Rubber as a Selective Barrier" in Industrial and Engineering Chemistry during 1957. The very high permeability of the silicone films, especially compared with materials previously available, coupled with what was known about optimum geometries resulted in a number of lasting device designs introduced in the early 1960's. The commercial availablity of microporous polyolefins and perfluoro-polyolefins in the 1970's followed with the introduction of membrane oxygenator devices using these materials. Note that with possible exception of silicone passivated, microporous cellulose acetate (the Rhone-Poulenc lung), no polymeric material in any commercial artificial lung was especially designed for the purpose of blood oxygenation. However, two polymers, ethyl-cellulose perfluorobutyrate (EFB) and the poly (alkyl sulfones) have been especially developed since the mid 1970's as the base for membranes for blood oxygenators. Ethyl cellulose perfluorobutyrate was developed by Northstar Research. The poly (alkyl sulfones) were developed by Owens-Illinois and are now offered under the BIOBLAND name by Shenandoah Research, Inc. While the materials have not yet been used commercially in devices, considerable evaluation and testing on these materials has been reported (Refs. 7 and 9 and pertinent references cited therein).

The early experimental devices were gradually improved by

Table I Permeability of various polymers to oxygen and carbon dioxide

	Polymer	P_{O_2}	P_{CO_2}
	Polydimethyl siloxane	500	2700
	Silicone rubber/polycarbonate copolymer (MEM 213)	160	970
Post 1955	Poly (alpha-hexadecene sulfone) (Biobland-16)	60	250
	Ethylcellulose perfluorobutyrate (EFB)	50	250
	Poly (4-methylpentene-1) (TPX)	30	90
	Poly (tetrafluoroethylene) (Teflon)	5	13
	Polypropylene (density 0.91)	2	9
	Polyethylene (density 0.96)	0.4	1.8
Pre 1955	Cellulose acetate (unplasticized)	0.08	0.016
	Polyvinylchloride (unplasticized)	0.045	0.016
	Polyethylene terephthalate-oriented (Mylar)	0.035	0.017

Units = $\dfrac{cm^3 \text{ (STP), cm}}{cm^2 \text{ ,sec, cm Hg}} \times 10^{10}$

Registered Trademarks

MEM 213 - General Electric
Biobland - 16 - Shenandoah Research Inc.
TPX - Mitsui
Teflon , Mylar - DuPont

Table II Significant milestones: Development of artificial membrane lungs

	CLINICAL ADVANCE	MATERIAL	TYPE		MATERIAL ADVANCE
				1943	First silicone production Dow-Corning
1944	Kolff & Berk note blood oxygenation in early renal dialysis trials	Regenerated cellulose (Cellophane)	'Hydrated' microporous		
1944	Kolff & Berk construct coil type membrane oxygenator	'Plastic' coated fiber-glass fabric	Permselective		
				1946	High pressure (LD) polyethylene
				1947	GE silicone production
				1950's	Teflon becomes available
1954	Successful heart surgery using cross circulation - (Lillehei)				
1955	Kolff & Balzar report on coil configuration polyethylene based oxygenator	LDPE?	Permselective		
				1955	Low pressure (HD) polyethylene available
1955-1956	Both bubble and disc types oxygenator used for heart surgery			1955-1956	Kammermeyer gets first silicone membrane from GE and determines permeability
1956	Clowes, Hopkins and Neville construct and test plate type oxygenator	Ethyl cellulose and Teflon	Permselective		
1963-1968	Bramson, Kolobow, Landé, Pierce and others contribute to membrane lung design	Mostly silicones and silicone polymers	Permselective	1962-1963	Poly (4-methyl pentene-1) available (TPX)
1973	Bellhouse — secondary flow design improves efficiency		Permselective	1972-1973	Microporous polypropylene (Celgard) becomes available
				1976	Microporous Teflon (Gore-Tex) becomes available
1978	Membrane lungs using microporous membranes introduced	Microporous materials	Microporous		

optimizing membrane material and flow characteristics, and by the early 1970's sufficient experimental data was available to indicate that membrane oxygenators were less damaging to blood than the blood-gas direct contact type (disc and bubble). Therefore, the newer blood oxygenators could be used for longer periods[8,9].

The improvements made in materials and oxygenator designs allowed clinicians to consider long-term (days rather than hours) oxygenation for the first time. Here again the hope was to "buy time" not for surgery, but for an injured or diseased lung to repair itself or heal. The workers developing these techniques were using as a model a well-proven extracorporeal technique - temporary dialysis with the artificial kidney. A distinct difference between renal dialysis and long-term oxygenation is that renal dialysis may be intermittent and still be effective, while oxygenation must be continuous in order to be effective. This requirement puts greater demands on the reliability of the support devices. As natural healing often did not occur despite buying time with artificial lungs, physicians have now turned their thoughts to using artificial lungs as support or replacement devices for insufficient natural lungs.

Materials used for the gas transfer membrane in artificial lungs can be of two types, permselective such as those previously discussed or microporous. In either case, gas passage properties must be high, blood compatibility must be optimal and toxic agents must not be released from the membranes. Zapol and Ketteringham[7] give the following characteristics required for membrane materials for an artificial lung:
1. They must have high oxygen and carbon dioxide permeability.
2. They should be chemically stable without leachable moieties and be blood compatible, minimizing thrombosis, platelet activation and injury, and protein denaturation.
3. They must be strong, pinhole-free and capable of withstanding a pressure gradient of 15 psi from the blood side without leaking.
4. They must be capable of sterilization preferably by ethylene oxide or by autoclaving.
5. They should be easily fabricated into pinhole-free membranes (containing a supporting component if necessary) with a surface conformation which can be designed to augment secondary blood flow against the surface.
6. The basic cost of the material and ease of fabrication must permit economical disposable devices to be constructed.

A number of configurations are used for commercial membrane lungs; those based on flat sheets are Bramson, G.E.-Pierce, Lande-Edwards and Travenol. A modification of the flat sheet configuration is the Kolobow/Sci-Med spiral coil membrane lung. Hollow fiber membrane lungs are represented by the Dow and the Terumo artificial lungs.

Blood flowing past a membrane, at least as the fluid velocities permitted in membrane lungs, forms a laminar boundary layer adjacent to the membrane. This phenomena limits the gas transfer properties, expecially oxygen, of the device. To exploit the true, high potential gas transfer capabilities of the membrane material in modern membrane lungs, Bellhouse and coworkers[11] have investigated vortex shedding, secondary flow techniques to increase membrane to blood gas transfer. This is accomplished by impressing a secondary pulsitile flow on the circulatory flow to disturb the laminar layer. Examples of devices using this technique are the Oxford pulsed flat sheet lung and the device offered by Extracorporeal. These devices that augment mixing and increase gas transfer per unit area have caused a re-evaluation of the membrane materials used in artificial lungs.

Ketteringham, deFilippi and Birkett[12] working with a number of permselective materials fabricated into ultrathin membranes have determined the CO_2/O_2 flux ratio from in vitro measurements using a series of artificial lungs with increasingly more efficient oxygen transfer characteristics. As can be seen from Table 1, for the polymers that are serious candidates as membranes, the carbon dioxide permeability is much higher than the oxygen permeability. In devices without induced or augmented secondary flow, the membrane area required to maintain adequate oxygen transfer to the blood was more than adequate for carbon dioxide clearance. With more efficient devices that eliminate or reduce the deleterious stagnant blood layer, the membrane area required for CO_2 clearance is also of concern. Figure 3 represents a simplified presentation of the information reported by Ketteringham[12]. The ratio CO_2 flux/O_2 flux is plotted versus the total oxygen flux. At a flux ratio less than 0.82, insufficient CO_2 is cleared relative to oxygen transfer. Therefore, any further improvement in total oxygen transfer is of no physiological advantage. The intercept of the curved lines with the dotted line yields the value for the highest usable O_2 transfer for a given material. BIOBLAND 16 used in the ultrathin membrane configuration approaches the gas transfer characteristics of the microporous materials, but without the problems associated with the microporous materials. The problems most often associated with the microporous membranes are possible blood damage due to gas microbubble intrusion, excessive water flux and possible seepage.

Since membrane lungs as extracorporeal devices are in wide use, thoughts have turned to an implantable artificial lung prosthesis based on membrane technology. Developing such a device with the adequate characteristics and long-term reliability is a much more difficult task than encountered with the extracorporeal device developed for intermittant use. However, a small prototype device made of porous Teflon has been fabricated and tested by Richardson and Galletti[13].

The hopes for the use of Extracorporeal Membrane Oxygenation (ECMO) for treating acute respiratory failure went through a low point in the mid 1970's after the results of the National Insti-

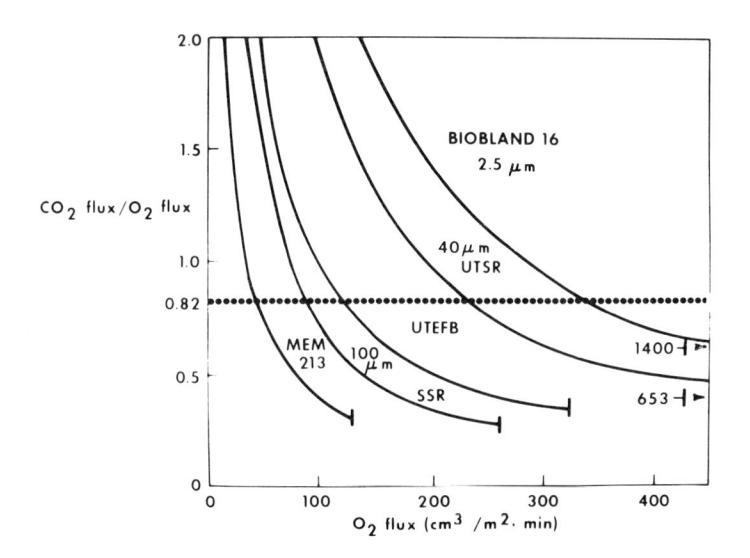

Figure 3. Membrane efficiencies. Key: MEM 213, polysiloxane/polycarbonate; SSR, standard silicone rubber; UTEFB, ultrathin ethyl cellulose perfluorobutyrate; UTSR, ultrathin silicone rubber; and BIOBLAND 16, poly(α-hexadecene sulfone). (Reproduced with permission from Ref. 12. Copyright 1976, Academic Press.)

tutes of Health-Extracorporeal Membrane Oxygenation study became known[14]. This work describes the findings of a cooperative study involving nine prominent medical centers well versed in expracorporeal perfusion. Ninety individuals were chosen whose condition (respiratory failure) offered them only a ten percent chance of survival using standard respiratory therapy management. This group was randomly divided into two smaller, equal groups (45 each), one group being given ECMO state-of-the-art support and the other given standard therapy. There were four (4) survivors in each group indicating that the more difficult and expensive ECMO therapy apparently yielded no benefits.

However, the gloomy prospect has brightened in the last five years. In 1979 Bartlett[15] reported on the survival of one-half of a group of 32 moribund infants using ECMO techniques and stated as a result of his findings that "recovery and survival should be routine if ECMO is instituted in the first two days of life".

As early as 1978, Kolobow[16] reported carbon dioxide could be removed from blood (and hence blood pH could be properly maintained) by shunting only 10-30% of the cardiac output through a membrane lung. This study has been followed by more clinical work by Kolobow and his associates[17,18]. In one study a 63% survival rate was obtained by simultaneously using ECMO for carbon dioxide removal coupled with classical ventilator techniques for oxygenation. These studies have prompted a reappraisal of the use of ECMO therapy with renewed emphasis on patient choice and modified treatment techniques.

It is expected that with the greater availability of simpler, more dependable and lower cost disposable membrane oxygenators in surgical procedures of the heart, their use will increase. In this country, about 500 individuals each day undergo routine heart surgery that requires extracorporeal oxygenation[22]. Bubble oxygenators still dominate, but the number of perfusion teams that are shifting to membrane units is increasing[23]. The total potential market (U.S.) for membrane lungs is about $20 million/year (at the present price of $200/unit) making it a relatively small market as compared, for example, to the artificial kidney (dialysis) market of $225 million/year. Therefore, one would not expect to see many new "me-too" membrane oxygenator devices introduced. Any new product would have to offer a clear benefit or fill a recognized need to capture market share.

Literature Cited

1. Galletti, P.M., Artificial Lungs for Acute Respiratory Failure, edited by Warren M. Zapol and Jesper Qvist, Academic Press (1976)
2. Lillehei, C.W., DeWall, R.A., Read, R.C., Warden, H.E. and Varco, R.L., Dis. Chest, 29, 1 (1956)
3. Kirklin, J.W., DuShane, J.W., Patrick, R.T., Donald, D.E., Hetzel, P.S., Harshbarger, H.G. and Wood, E.H., Proc. Staff Meet., Mayo Clin, 30, 201 (1955)
4. Kolff, W.J. and Balzer, R., Trans. Am. Soc. Artif. Intern. Organs, 1, 39 (1955)
5. Clowes, G.H., Jr., Hopking, A.L. and Neville, W.E., J. Thoracic Surg., 32, 630 (1956)
6. Private Communication - Prof. Sun-Tak Hwang, University of Cincinnati
7. Kammermeyer, K., Ind. and Eng. Chem., 49, 1685-1686 (1957)
8. Lande, A.J., Fillmore, S.J., Subramanian, V., Tiedenamm, R.N., Carlson, R.G., Bloch, J.A. and Lillehei, C.W., Trans. Soc. Artif. Intern. Organs, 15, 181 (1969)
9. Kolobow, T. and Zapol, W.M., Adv. Cardiol., 6, 112 (1971)
10. Zapol, W.M. and Ketteringham, J.M., Polymers in Medicine and Surgery, Polymer Science and Technology, Volume 8, Plenum Press, N.Y. (1975)
11. Bellhouse, B.J., Bellhouse, F.M., Curl, C.M., MacMillan, T.I., Gunning, A.J., Spratt, E.M., MacMurray, S.B. and Nelems, J.M., Trans. Am. Soc. Artif. Intern. Organs, 19, 72 (1973)
12. Ketteringham, J.M., DeFillippi, R. and Birkett, J.D., Ultrathin Membranes for Membrane Lungs, in Artificial Lungs for Acute Respiratory Failure, Zapol, W.M. and J. Qvist, ed., Academis Press (1976)
13. Galletti, P.M., Richardson, P.D., Trudell, L.A., Parol, G., Tanishita, K. and Accinelli, D., Trans. Am. Soc. Artif. Intern. Organs, 26, 573 (1980)
14. Zapol, W., Snider, M.T., Hill, J.D., Fallat, R.J., Bartlett, R.H., Edmunds, L.H., Morris, A.H., Pierce, E.C., II, Thomas, A.N., Drinker, P.A., Pratt, P.C., Bagiewski, A., Miller, R.G. Jr., Extracorporeal membrane oxygenation in severe acute respiratory failure. A randomized prospective study. JAMA 242, 2193 (1979)
15. Bartlett, R.H., Gazzaniga, A.B., Huxtable, R.H., Rucker, R., Wetmore, N., Haiduc, N. Extracorporeal membrane oxygenation (EMCO) in newborn respiratory failure: Technical considerations. Trans. Am. Soc. Artif. Intern. Organs, 25, 473 (1979)
16. Kolobow, T. Gattinoni, L., Tomlinson, T., Pierce, J.E., An alternative to breathing. J. Thorac. Cardiovasc. Surg., 75, 261 (1978)
17. Gattinoni, L., Pesenti, A., Pelizzola, A., Caspani, M.L., Iapichino, G., Agostoni, A., Damia, G., and Kolobow, T., Reversal of terminal acute respiratory failure by low

frequency positive pressure ventilation with extracorporeal removal of CO_2 (LFPPV-ECCO$_2$R). Trans. Am. Soc. Artif. Intern. Organs, 27, 289 (1981)
18. Pesenti, A., Pelizzola, A., Mascheroni, D., Uziel, L, Pirovani, E., Fox, U., Gattinoni, L. and Kolobow, T., Low frequency positive pressure ventilation with extracorporeal CO_2 removal (LFPPV-ECCO$_2$R) in acute respiratory failure (ARF); Technique. Trans. Am. Soc. Artif. Intern. Organs, 27, 263 (1981)
19. Warden, H.E., Cohen, M., DeWall, R.A., Schultz, E.A., Buckley, J.J., Read, R.C., Lillehei, C.W. Experimental closure of intraventricular septal defects and further physiologic studies on controlled cross circulation. Surg. Forum, 5, 22 (1954)
20. Warden, H.E., Cohen, M. Read, R.C., Lillehei, C.W. Controlled cross circulation for open intracardiac surgery. J. Thorac. Surg., 28, 331 (1954)
21. Campbell, G.S., Crisp, N.W., Brown, E.B. Total cardiac bypass in humans utilizing a pump and heterologous lung oxygenator (dog lungs). Surgery, 40, 364 (1956)
22. Gott, V.L., Extracorporeal Circulation: 1970-1982, Trans. Am. Soc. Artif. Inter. Organs, 28, 17 (1982)
23. Galletti, P.M., Impact of the artificial lung on medical care, Int. J. of Artif. Organs, 3, 157 (1980)

RECEIVED March 19, 1984

Blood Compatibility of Artificial Organs
Transient Leukopenia in Hemodialysis

S. MURABAYASHI and Y. NOSE

Department of Artificial Organs, Cleveland Clinic Foundation, Cleveland, OH 44106

> Blood compatible materials are essential for artificial organs which are used in contact with blood. The immunological aspects of blood compatibility are stressed. Complement activation induced by material-blood interaction is most likely related to transient leukopenia during extracorporeal circulation such as hemodialysis. Although transient, it may be harmful, especially if it occurs frequently. Some complications associated with hemodialysis may be caused due to the repeated complement activation and leukostasis in the lung. Cellulosic membranes induce the phenomenon more severely than synthetic membranes. Reused cellulosic membranes sterilized with aldehyde after the first use show less complement activation and leukopenia. Aldehyde treated biological substances may play a important role in enhancing blood compatibility. This concept is similar to our "Biolization" philosophy, which was proved in the cardiac prostheses. Transient leukopenia in hemodialysis was reviewed from a material blood compatibility point of view.

For the past three decades, technological advances have revolutionized the field of artificial organs. Various devices have prolonged the lives of millions of persons and improvements are still continuing for the benefits of the patient. The material used in artificial organs is an important factor contributing to the good performance of the device. The choice of materials is dependent upon both its biofunctionality and biocompatibility. Biofunctionality includes the physical, chemical, and mechanical properties of the material, and relates to the intended performance of the item or devices. Ideally, the devices should function as originally intended throughout their entire usage period. Biocompatibility refers to the absence of any

0097-6156/84/0256-0163$06.00/0
© 1984 American Chemical Society

adverse effect that the material might present to the physiological system, in particular to the blood or natural tissue. In the early development of artificial organs, emphasis was placed primarily on the biofunctionality of the materials. In recent years, the emphasis has turned to the enhancement of the biocompatibility aspect.

In the composition of any device which contacts blood, blood compatibile materials are essential. While clotting and thrombosis are the most obvious evidence of incompatibility, they represent only one aspect of blood compatibility. Materials can affect the plasma proteins, clotting factors and immunological factors. As early as 20 years ago, changes in circulating blood cellular elements were noted during extracorporeal circulation (1). In these early studies, leukocyte counts decreased during the first 10-15 minutes of perfusion and then returned to near normal levels. Serum, taken from an animal on extracorporeal circulation and injected into a healthy animal resulted in decreases in circulatory polymorphonuclear leukocytes. Humoral factors activated or produced during extracorporeal circulation were thus implicated in these changes. In hemodialysis, this phenomenon, termed transient leukopenia, has been shown to occur in the early phase of the procedure. Immunological alterations induced by materials are taken into consideration recently, since transient leukopenia during hemodialysis is most likely related to complement activation when blood comes into contact with hemodialysis membranes. Immunological aspects of the membrane materials used in commercial dialyzers are discussed by reviewing the transient leukopenia observed during hemodialysis.

Leukopenia in Hemodialysis

Profound transient leukopenia during hemodialysis with cellophane membranes was first published in English by Kaplow and Goffinet (2). The fall in circulating leukocytes was due almost entirely to a reduction in the number of circulating neutrophilic granulocytes and occurred during the first 15 minutes of dialysis. No striking changes were noted in platelet or erythrocyte levels. The leukocyte count returns to normal levels one hour after the start of dialysis. This phenomenon is not associated with chills or fever. Since this early report in 1968, many instances have been noted. Although large numbers of granulocytes adhere to the dialysis cellophane membrane, the absolute number lost cannot account for the fall in leukocyte count (1, 3,). Evidence from studies in dialyzed dogs suggests that this leukopenia is the result of cell sequestration within the pulmonary vasculature (4). This sequestration is transient, followed by return of the trapped leukocytes to the circulation within 1-2 hours, and accompanied by cells released from the bone marrow storage pool (5). Simple withdrawl and reinfusion of blood does not appreciably affect the neutrophil count (3), nor will

administration of heparin (2), exposure blood to intravenous
tubing (2), or infusion of saline or albumin exposed to dialysis
coil cause neutropenia (6). This phenomenon occurs with coil,
parallel plate and hollow fiber type cellulosic membrane dialyzers
(7) and is not related to the method of sterilization (7). If
heparinized human plasma is exposed to dialyzer cellophane and
reinfused into human, it induced the acute transient leukopenia.
These data suggests that some plasma factors which are activated
by contact with dialyzer cellophane induce pulmonary leukostasis
and the consequent leukopenia. Although this phenomenon is
recognized to be related to the cellulosic membrane, it was not
considered seriously in the treatment of patients, since it was a
transient phenomenon and there was no other material available
except cellulosic membrane for the hemodialyzer at that time.
However, in recent years with the introduction of synthetic
membrane which do not induce profound leukopenia, this phenomenon
is taken into consideration with respect to the mechanism induced
and its influences on uremic patients undergoing chronic
maintenance hemodialysis. Although transient, this pulmonary
leukostasis may be harmful, especially if it occurs frequently. A
pulmonary fibrosis-calcinosis syndrome, which develops in many
patients given long-term hemodialysis treatments (8), may reflect
injury caused by repeated plugging of the microvasculature by
leukocytes.

Possible Mechanisms In Transient Leukopenia

Plasma factors which might be responsible for the phenomenon
were suggested by Craddock et al (9, 10). They demonstrated that
dialyzer Cuprophane activated complement through alternative
pathway both in vitro and in hemodialysis patients, and proposed
that activation of complement would lead to intravascular
granulocyte aggregates that are entrapped in the lung. They
showed that reinfusion of autologous, Cuprophane incubated plasma
into rabbits produced selective neutropenia identical to that
seen in dialyzed patients. Lungs from such animals revealed
striking pulmonary vessel engorgement with granulocytes. Infusion
of plasma in which complement was activated by zymosan incubation
also produced a similar neutropenia. In contrast no leukostasis
was observed when plasma was heated at $56°C$ to prevent complement
activation before Cuprophane incubation. Addition of EDTA
(ethylenediaminetetracetic acid) to plasma before Cuprophane
incubation prevented neutropenia, whereas EGTA
(ethyleneglycoltetracetic acid)/Mg^{2+} which selectively inhibits
activation of the classical pathway was noninhibitory. Moreover,
immunoelectrophoretic analysis of serum from dialysis patients
revealed the conversion of both C_3 and factor B during the first
hour of each dialysis, and simple incubation of human plasma with
Cuprophane caused identical complement activation.

Based upon this evidence, Craddock reasoned that

granulocyte sequestration might result from either or both of two mechanisms: 1) Complement - mediated adhesion of individual granulocytes to the vascular endothelium, or 2) Complement - induced granulocyte aggregation in the circulation with pulmonary embolization of the aggregates so formed. Sephadex - fractionation of Cuprophane incubated rabbit plasma revealed that the margination - inducing complement fragment was of a molecular weight of 7000-20,000 daltons similar to that of C5a or C3a (9). They suggested that C5a might be responsible for the leukopenia, since it can induce neutrophilic auto-aggregation (11), and plasma from genitically C5 deficient donors was incapable of producing granulocyte aggregation in vitro.

Recently, a component of C3 activation, namely C3e which is a fragment of the α chain of C3, has been found to induce in rabbits an initial leukopenia at 15-30 minutes after infusion, followed by leukocytosis, which reaches a maximum at 12 hours (12). Although the presence of C3e fragments has not been demonstrated during dialysis, it is very interesting that C3e showed the capability of producing leukocytosis. C5a has neutropenia inducing activity, but it has not been reported to produce leukocytosis which occurs during hemodialysis followed by leukopenia.

TABLE I: EFFECT OF DIFFERENT MEMBRANES ON LEUKOPENIA AND ACTIVATION OF COMPLEMENT

Membrane	Complement Activation	Leukopenia	Ref.
Cellophane	+++	+++	14-16
Cuprophane	+++	+++	13-16
Polycarbonate	+	++	13
Polyacrylonitrile	++	+	13,14,16
Polymethylmethacrylate	+	+	15,16
Cellulose acetate		+	14,16
Polyethylvinyl alcohol		++	16

Inspired by reports from Craddok, the effects of different membranes on hemodialysis induced leukopenia and complement activation were studied (Table I). The results were disappointing. There was no definite correlation between the reduction in neutrophil count and complement activation. Unfortunately, however, these studies did not include a measure of complement split products. Serum hemolytic complement assays were performed to evaluate the consumption of complement. Since complement component levels represent a dynamic balance between synthesis and degradation of components, their assay will fail to detect a state of increased complement consumption, if such consumption is balanced by an increased synthesis (17).

Nonetheless, it is interesting to note that component depletion of complement is not associated with neutropenia. This explanation remains unclear and further investigations are expected to answer these problems.

Complications Associated With Transient Leukopenia

Although transient leukopenia during hemodialysis was noted as early as 20 years ago, its influence on a patient was not seriously considered. This phenomenon was regarded as relatively harmless to a patient, since it was transient and not associated with any severe complications. However, as the mechanism is becoming understood, complications which might be related to the transient leukopenia will be discussed.

Dialysis patients seem prone to bacterial infection and infection is the principal cause of the hospitalization of chronic renal failure patients. Complement activation with repeated dialysis may potentially lead to depletion of complement components. Zeig (18) and Myers (19) observed depressed levels of C3 in chronic hemodialysis patients and suggested that this may predispose them to bacterial infection. The cyclic variation of the number and function of neutrophils with each dialysis and the decreased chemotactic responsiveness may also contribute to the high level of infection. Henderson et al found significant decreases in phagocytosis and random mobility when neutrophils were exposed to cellulosic membrane (20). Lespier-Dexter et al evaluated granulocyte adherence in uremia and hemodialysis patients and demonstrated that patients undergoing hemodialysis had significant impairment of granulocyte function (21).

With regard to the influence of leukostasis in the lung, Craddock et al suggested that dialysis-induced hypoxia may reflect the complement-mediated pulmonary leukostasis (10). Aljama et al reported a patient in whom hemodialysis with a Cuprophan membrane was associated with severe asthma (22). Dramatic improvement was observed when the Cuprophane membrane was substituted with polyacrylonitrile membrane which does not cause appreciable leukopenia. Jacob suspected that the pulmonary fibrosis/calcinosis syndrome that is seen in long term hemodialysis patients may reflect the repeated endothelial damage that occurs with each dialysis (23). A high-protein, intestitial pulmonary edema forms in dialyzed sheep which suggests pulmonary endothelial damage (10). Indeed, such endothelial damage was demonstrated to occur when cultured endothelial cells are exposed to granulocytes plus C5, but not to either when they are added alone (24). In these in vitro studies, the damaging substances that are released from the triggered granulocytes appear mainly consisting of toxic substances such as O_2^- and H_2O_2. Repeated production of these substances, which were reported to inhibit platelet function, may be related to the hemorrhagic tendency in patients undergoing hemodialysis (25).

Reuse of Dialyzer and "Biolization" Concept

Dialyzer reuse has become common practice because of financial constraints. Approximately 17% of all hemodialysis in the United States was performed by reused dialyzer in 1981, and the proportion of reused dialyzers is increasing. Recent evidence suggests that the reuse of dialyzers may lead to significant medical benefits. A survey by Wing et al involving a large number of patients in the United Kingdom showed a significant decrease of mortality in patients reusing dialyzers (26). Kant and Pollack showed that adverse symptoms such as chest pain, respiratory distress and cramps were significantly less frequent with reuse than with first use (27). Hakim and Lowrie studied effect of dialyzer reuse on leukopenia and complement system, and demonstrated reuse of cellulosic membrane dialyzer leads a significant decrease in the extent of complement activation and leukopenia (15). This evidence reveals that reuse of dialyzers improve the blood compatibility. The questions may be asked, then why? In preparation for the reuse, formaldehyde solution is used for disinfectant purposes, after rinsing the dialyzer with saline. When a dialyzer membrane comes in contact with blood at the first use, they become coated with plasma proteins or other blood components. These substances remain on the surface even after rinsing with saline. Therefore, blood contacting surfaces of the reused dialyzer is not the native cellulose, but biological substances treated with formaldehyde. Thus, the improvement of blood compatibility was achieved by aldehyde treated biological substances. This concept is similar to our hypothesis termed "Biolization", to produce blood compatabile materials. The hypothesis mentions that following two-step process would promote thromboresistance and biocompatibility of any materials (28).

1) Activation by a biological substances, such as protein or polysaccaride, and
2) Biological inactivation by aldehyde, heat or other treatment.

Since 1970 biolized materials have been utilized in our cardiac prostheses. Long term survival of TAH (total artificial heart) and LVAD (left ventricular assist device) implanted in animals has shown successful application of these materials without the use of anticoagulants (29).

Concluding Remarks

Transient leukopenia by complement activation during hemodialysis was described in this article. Complement activation and pulmonary leukostasis have been also observed during filtration leukapheresis (30) and cardiopulmonary bypass (31).

Such immunological alterations induced by materials are now recognized as one of the important aspects of blood compatibility. When materials come in contact with blood, they can affect plasma proteins and cells, clotting factors and immunological factors, and induce adverse reactions in the body. Even though most of these reactions might be tolerated by the body, it is important to minimize them. Evidences such as the enhanced blood compatibility of reused dialyzers and good performance in our blood pumps suggest that the "Biolization" concept would be one possible approach to the development of biocompatibile materials.

Literature Cited

1. Mito, Y.; Nishimura, A.; Sumiyoshi, A.; Kawai, M.; Nose, Y.; Kawamura, Y.; Yoshimoto, C.; Sogoigaku 1960, 17, 86.
2. Kaplow, L.S.; Goffinet, J.A.; JAMA 1968, 203, 1135.
3. Buscarini, L.; Bassi, F.; Acta Haematol. 1972, 48 278.
4. Toren, M.; Goffinet, JA.; Kaplow, L.S. Blood 1970, 36, 337.
5. Brubaker, L.H.; Nolph, K.D. Blood 1971, 38, 623.
6. Jensen, D.P.; Brubaker, L.H.; Nolph, K.D.; Johnson, C.A.; Nothum, R.J.; Blood 1973, 41, 399.
7. Gral, T.; Schroth, P.; Depalma, J.R.; Gordon, A. Trans. Am. Soc. Artif. Intern. Organs 1969, 14. 45
8. Conger, J.D.; Hammond, W.S.; Alfrey, A.C.; Contiguglia, S.R.; Stanford, R.E.; Huffer, W.E. Ann. Intern. Med. 1975, 83, 330.
9. Craddock, P.R.; Fehr, J.; Dalmasso, A.P.; Brigham, K.L.; Jacob, H.S. J. Clin. Invest. 1977, 59, 879.
10. Craddock, P.R.; Fehr, J.; Brigham, K.L.; Kranenberg, R.S.; Jacob, H.S. N. Engl. J. Med. 1977, 296, 769.
11. Craddock, P.R.; Hammerschmidt, D.; White, J.G.; Dalmasso, A.P.; Jacobs, H.S. J. Clin. Invest. 1977, 60, 260.
12. Ghebrehiwet, G.; Muller-Eberhard, HJ. J. Immunol. 1979, 123, 616.
13. Aljama, P.; Bird, P.A.E.; Ward, M.K.; Feest, T.G.; Walker, W.; Tanboga, H.; Sussman, M.; Kerr, D.N.S. Proc. Eur. Dial. Transplant. Assoc. 1978, 15, 144.
14. Jacob, A.I.; Gavellas, G.; Zarco, R.; Perez, G.; Bourgoignie, J.J. Kidney Intern. 1980, 18, 606.
15. Hahim, R.M.; Lowrie, E.G. Trans. Am. Soc. Artif. Intern. Organs 1980, 26, 159.
16. Shin, J.; Matsuo, M.; Shinko, S.; Fujita, Y.; Inoue, S.; Sakai, R.; Nishioka, N. J. Dial. 1980, 4, 51.
17. Hammerschmidt, D.E.; Bowers, T.K.; Lammi-Keefe, C.J.; Jacobs, H.S.; Craddock, P.R. Blood 1980, 55, 898.
18. Zeig, S.; Paran, E.; Freidman, E.A.; Berlyne, G.M. Artificial Organs 1978, (S)2, 450.

19. Myer, B.D.; Klajman, A. Israel. J. Med. Sci. 1975, 11, 335.
20. Henderson, L.W.; Miller, M.E.; Hamilton, R.W.; Norman, M.E. J. Lab. Clin. Med. 1975, 85, 191.
21. Lespier-Dexter, L.E.; Guerra, C.; Ojeda, W.; Martinez-Maldonado, M. Nephron. 1979, 24, 64.
22. Aljama, P.; Brown, P.; Turner, P.; Ward, MK.; Kerr, D.N.S. Br. Med. J. 1978, 22, 251.
23. Jacob, H.S. Arch. Intern. Med. 1978, 138, 461.
24. Sacks, T.; Maldow, C.F.; Craddock, P.R.; Jacobs, H.S. Clin. Res. 1977, 25, 347a.
25. Levine, P.H.; Weinger, R.S.; Simon, J.; Scoon, K.L.; Krinsky, N.I. J. Clin. Invest. 1976, 57, 955.
26. Wing, A.J.; Brunner, F.P.; Brynger, H.A.O.; Chantler, C.; Donckerwolcke, RA.; Gurland, H.J.; Jacobs, C.; Selwood, N.H. Br. Med. J. 1978, 23, 853.
27. Kant, K.S.; Pollak, V.E. Chronic Renal Disease Conference (NIAMDO) 1980, p. 33.
28. Nose, Y.; Tajima, K.; Imai, Y.; Klain, M.; Mrava, G.; Schriber, K.; Urbanek, K.; Ogawa, H. Trans. Am. Soc. Artif. Intern. Organs 1971, 17, 482.
29. Kambic, H.E.; Murabayashi, S.; Nose, Y. "Biocompatible Polymers: Science and Technology"; Szycher M., Ed. Technomic Publishing Co., Lancaster, 1982, p. 179.
30. Hammerschmidt, D.E.; Craddock, P.R.; McCullough, J.; Kronenberg, RS.; Dalmasso, A.P.; Jacob, H.S. Blood 1978, 51, 721.
31. Kolobow, T.; Tomlinson, T.; Pierce, J.; Gattinoni, L.; Trans. Am. Soc. Artif. Intern. Organs 1976, 22, 110.

RECEIVED April 23, 1984

Artificial Cells

THOMAS MING SWI CHANG

Artificial Cells and Organs Research Centre, McGill University, Faculty of Medicine, 3655 Drummond St., Montreal, PQ, Canada H3G 1Y6

Artificial cells were first prepared in 1957. Since then, there has been increasing basic, applied and clinical research in this area. At present, artificial cells are being investigated clinically as blood substitutes; artificial kidney; detoxifier; artificial liver; drug carriers; immunosorbent; hemoperfusion and other areas. They are also being investigated for their applications in biotechnology in the areas of immobilized enzymes, biologicals, and cells.

Since artificial cells were first prepared by the author in 1957 [1,2] an increasing number of approaches to their use are now available. Thus, artificial cell membranes can now be formed using a variety of synthetic or biological materials, resulting in variations of permeability, surface properties and blood compatibility. Almost any material can be included within artificial cells. These include enzyme systems, cell extracts, biological cells, magnetic material, isotopes, antigens, antibodies, vaccines, hormones, adsorbents and others. A number of potential applications, suggested earlier, have now reached the clinical trial or clinical application stage. Detailed reviews are available [4-7].

RED BLOOD CELL SUBSTITUTE

Since 1956 we have investigated the feasibility of using artificial red blood cells for use in blood transfusion [1-3]. Initially, we prepared artificial cells in the form of microencapsulated hemoglobin. In-vitro, these artificial cells did not interact with blood group antibodies, but they could transport oxygen and carbon dioxide. However, after infusion, they were removed rapidly from the circulation.

We also prepared artificial red blood cells with an organic material, silicone rubber, as the major component [8,9]. Silicone rubber microspheres can transport oxygen. However, they were removed rapidly from the circulation. Other groups were testing a similar material in the form of silicone oil and fluorocarbon fluid for transporting of oxygen. Later, they prepared a fine emulsion of fluorocarbon oil as a red blood cell substitute [10]. By coating the surface with phospholipids to form an artificial cell membrane, the fluorocarbon emulsion could become stabiilized and blood compatible. Clinical trials have been initiated in Japan and U.S.A. However the long-term in-vivo effects of fluorocarbon are not known.

We earlier demonstrated that hemoglobin could be cross-linked by using a bifunctional agent, forming a large polyhemoglobin. This permitted the artificial cells to be made much smaller than microencapsulated hemoglobin [2-4,9]. This has now been developed further so that hemoglobin can be cross-linked into an even smaller polyhemoglobin which remains in solution. Studies, being carried out at this Research Centre, have shown that the small polyhemoglobin survived much longer in the circulation, as compared to stroma-free hemoglobin [11].

THE ROLE OF ARTIFICIAL CELLS IN ARTIFICIAL ORGANS

The rate of equilibration in 10 ml of 20 µ diameter artificial cells is 400 times higher than for a standard hemodialysis machine [3,5,8]. Furthermore, membrane properties of artificial cells can be varied over a wide range to allow for changes in permeability characteristics and surface properties. The very small volume of artificial cells required, and the variations possible, result in different types of miniaturized artificial organs. Both theoretical analyses and animal studies have demonstrated the feasibility of using the principle of artificial cells to form extremely compact, efficient and simple artificial organs. By varying the contents of the artificial cells (adsorbents, detoxicants, enzymes, cell extracts, cells and other biologically active materials), the artificial organs can be adjusted to carry out different biochemical or detoxification functions. The principle of artificial cells has already been used to form blood compatible charcoal and resin hemoperfusion systems for use in patients, as a blood detoxifier (poisoning), artificial kidney, artificial liver, or immunosorbent. These will be described below.

ARTIFICIAL CELLS FOR ARTIFICIAL KIDNEY

The large surface to volume relationship and the ultrathin membrane allows rapid equilibration of metabolites into the artificial cells. By placing enzymes, ion exchange resin and activated charcoal inside artificial cells, it was demonstrated that the artificial cells could be used for hemoperfusion, a new form of artificial kidney [8]. The principle of artificial cells, containing activated charcoal for hemoperfusion, was developed further to a stage for clinical application [12,13]. In treating uremic patients, we have reported improvements in nausea, vomiting, pruritis, feeling of well-being, and in peripheral neuropathy [14,15]. This approach is much more efficient in removing organic uremic waste metabolites than standard hemodialysis. However, it does not remove water, electrolytes or urea. As a result, hemoperfusion has been combined in series with hemodialysis. This approach solves the problems of electrolyte, urea and fluid removal [16]. We initially demonstrated that a 2-hour ACAC hemoperfusion-hemodialysis can replace 6 hours of standard hemodialysis. Furthermore, this approach resulted in improvements in nerve conduction velocity. This has stimulated interest in this combined approach and, in the most recent large-scale studies carried out in Italy, the effectiveness of this approach has been clearly demonstrated [17]. Another approach is the combined use of hemoperfusion and a small (0.2 m^2) ultrafiltrator, the latter for removal of water and sodium chloride [16]. In this approach, no hemodialysis equipment is required and the ultrafiltrator is used only to remove and discard all the filtered fluid (up to 2.7 liters), based entirely on the hydrostatic pressure controlled by the blood pump. A preliminary long-term clinical evaluation has demonstrated the safety and effectiveness of this approach [18]. The completion of this system will have to wait for the development of a urea removal system. Recently, a composite artificial kidney has been formed, combining artificial cells and dialysis or artificial cells and an ultrafiltrator [19].

ARTIFICIAL CELLS IN POISONING

Hemoperfusion, using artificial cells containing activated charcoal, is effective in treating severe acute drug poisoning for those drugs which can be adsorbed, and which have a small volume distribution [20]. High drug clearances have been obtained: glutethimide 230 ml/min, phenobarbital 228 ml/min, methyprylon 230 ml/min, methaqualone 230 ml/min, and secobarbital 200 ml/min. The effectiveness of hemoperfusion for those drugs with a high volume distribution, e.g., tricyclic antidepressants and digoxin, is still controversial.

This approach has also been used in the treatment of acute intoxication in pediatric patients [21]. The amberlite resin hemoperfusion system has a high clearance for many drugs [22]. However, the problem of platelet depletion was noted with this system. More recently, our approach of using an albumin-coating to make the particle surface more blood compatible for hemoperfusion [12] has been applied to the coating of resins. As a result, hemoperfusion with albumin-coated amberlite does not deplete platelets.

ARTIFICIAL CELLS AS ARTIFICIAL LIVER

Our initial observation that hemoperfusion can result in the temporary recovery of consciousness in grade IV hepatic coma patients [23] is now conclusively supported by other centers [5-7]. However, its effect on long-term survival has not yet been established. A galactosamine-induced fulminant hepatic coma rat model has been used to study in detail the effects of charcoal hemoperfusion on the survival rates of the animals [24-28]. ACAC hemoperfusion has been conclusively demonstrated to increase both survival time and survival rate of rats in the early stages of hepatic coma. ACAC hemoperfusions carried out in the later stage of hepatic coma increased the survival time but not the survival rate. The same results were obtained through homologous liver perfusion which increased the survival rate of rats in the early stages of hepatic coma, but not those in the later stage of coma. The present results would indicate that hemoperfusion plays an important role for the support of early stages of hepatic coma. In a later stage of coma, perhaps irreversible changes have already taken place. The results of experimental studies in animals from this laboratory [24-28] demonstrating the need for earlier treatment have now been corroborated by an initial clinical trial [29]. Thus, larger scale clinical trial is now ready to investigate this artificial liver concept further, based on artificial cells, for the treatment of patients in the earlier stages of fulminant hepatic failure [30].

We have also investigated the use of artificial cells containing tyrosinase to carry out some metabolic functions of the liver [31]. Results in animals show that tyrosinase artificial cells, retained in extracorporeal shunts perfused by blood, can effectively lower the systemic blood tyrosine levels of liver failure rats. Artificial cells, to carry out other metabolic functions of the liver, are also being studied. For instance, using artificial cells containing multienzyme systems with cofactor recycling [32], we have studied the *in-vitro* conversion of ammonia sequentially into different types of amino acids. This way, ammonia has been converted into glutamate and then sequentially into alanine or other amino acids.

ARTIFICIAL CELLS AND IMMUNOSORBENT

The ACAC hemoperfusion system developed by the author consists of albumin-collodion coated charcoal [12]. Albumin makes the surface blood compatible and also takes part in interacting with material in the circulating blood, including the facilitated transport of loosely protein-bound substances [5]. Terman reported the interesting finding that these ACAC microcapsules can also be used to remove antibodies to albumin from dog plasma [33]. He proceeded further to incorporate other types of antigens or antibodies onto the surface of this ACAC artificial cell system, resulting in immunosorbents for different types of applications. In very preliminary studies he found that, by replacing the albumin of the ACAC system with protein A for use in plasma perfusion, he was able to significantly reduce the size of breast carcinomas in patients.

Another area involves the use of synthetic immunosorbents. In order to prevent the problem of particulate release and blood incompatibility, we coated synthetic immunosorbents for blood group A & B with albumin and collodion. It was demonstrated that the synthetic immunosorbent could still remove the anti-A and anti-B blood group but did not affect platelets or release particulates [33]. An albumin-coated system has since been used clinically by another centre to remove anti-A and anti-B from plasma of patients prior to bone marrow transplantation.

ARTIFICIAL CELLS CONTAINING ENZYME SYSTEM

The injection of free enzyme of heterogenous origin may result in hypersensitivity reactions, production of antibodies, and rapid removal and inactivation. Furthermore, free enzymes cannot be kept at the desired sites of action and are less stable at a body temperature of 37°C. The use of artificial cells containing enzymes and proteins has been investigated [3,4]. Some examples of research being carried out will be briefly mentioned.

The first demonstration of the use of artificial cells for enzyme replacement in hereditary enzyme deficiency conditions involved the implantation of artificial cells containing catalase to replace the hereditary catalase deficiency in acatalasemic mice [3.4]. We have also demonstrated that artificial cells containing asparaginase are effective in the experimental suppression of lymphosarcoma in animal studies [3.4]. As described earlier, the feasibility of using artificial cells containing tyrosinase for the in-vivo conversion of tyrosine and phenols in fulminant hepatic failure rats has also been studied [31]. Our work in the area of artificial cells with cofactor recycling and multienzyme systems [4] led to the development of artificial cells containing multienzyme systems for sequential substrate conversion [32]. For instance, in the same artificial cell, urea can be converted by urease into ammonia; ammonia is then converted by glutamate dehydrogenase into glutamic acid; glutamic acid can be further converted by transaminase into other amino acids. The cofactor NADH required is recycled using glucose dehydrogenase or alcohol dehydrogenase. The cofactor can be retained within the artificial cells by covalent linkage to soluble macromolecules like dextrans [4] or by the use of artificial cells with lipid complexed membrane [35].

ARTIFICIAL CELLS CONTANING BIOLOGICAL CELLS

Artificial cells were prepared to contain biological cells [2,3]. We suggested that, this way, the microencapsulated biological cells, when implanted, can be separated from immunological rejection and proposed the use of this for the in-vivo implantation of endocrine cells [3]. A recent development has resulted in in-vivo experiments demonstrating that this suggestion is possible. For instance, rat-islet cells have been microencapsulated and then implanted intraperitoneally into diabetic rats [36]. In this way the microencapsulated islet cells can function to maintain normal glucose levels in the diabetic animals. Artificial cells containing fibroblasts or plasma cells have also been used in in-vitro tests for the production of interferon and monoclonal antibodies [37].

GENERAL DISCUSSION

The biological cell is the fundamental unit of all organs. It is thus not too surprising that its synthetic counterpart, the artificial cell, is playing an increasing role in artificial organs. The present paper only briefly describes a few examples to illustrate the application of artificial cells in medicine, biotechnology and other areas.

ACKNOWLEDGMENT

This research has been supported by the Medical Research Council of Canada and, at present, in the form of a special project grant (MRC-SP-4).

LITERATURE CITED

1. Chang, T.M.S., Hemoglobin corpuscles, report of research project for Honours B.Sc., McGill University, 1957.

2. Chang, T.M.S., Semipermeable microcapsules, Science, 146, 524, 1964.

3. Chang, T.M.S., Artificial Cells, Charles C. Thomas, Publisher, Springfield, Ill, 1972.

4. Chang, T.M.S., Biomedical Application of Immobilized Enzymes and Proteins, Vols. I & II, Plenum Press, New York, 1977.

5. Chang, T.M.S., Artificial Kidney, Artificial Liver, and Artificial Cells, Plenum Press, New York, 1978.

6. Sideman, S. and Chang, T.M.S., Hemoperfusion: Artificial Kidney and Liver Support and Detoxification, Part I, Hemisphere, Washington, D.C., 1980.

7. Bonomini, V. and Chang, T.M.S., Hemoperfusion, Contributions to Nephrology Series, S. Karger AG, Basel, 1982.

8. Chang, T.M.S., Semipermeable aqueous microcapsules ("artificial cells"): with emphasis on experiments in an extracorporeal shunt system, Trans. Amer. Soc. Artif. Internal Organs, 12, 13, 1966.

9. Chang, T.M.S., Artificial red blood cells, Trans. Amer. Soc. Artif. Internal Organs, 26, 354-357, 1980.

10. Mitsuno, T. and Naito, R., Perflurochemical Blood Substitutes, Excerpta Medica, Amsterdam, 1979, 469.

11. Keipert, P.M., Minkowitz, J. and Chang, T.M.S., Cross-linked stroma-free polyhemoglobin as a potential blood substitute. Int. J. Artif. Organs, 5, 383-385, 1982.

12. Chang, T.M.S., Removal of endogenous and exogenous toxins by a microencapsulated absorbent. Can. J. Physiol. Pharmacol., 47, 1043, 1969.

13. Chang, T.M.S. and Malave, N., The development and first clinical use of semipermeable microcapsules (artificial cells) as a compact artificial kidney. Trans. Amer. Soc. Artif. Internal Organs, 16, 141, 1970.

14. Chang, T.M.S., Gonda, A., Dirks, J.H. and Malave, N., Clinical evaluation of chronic intermittent or short-term hemoperfusions

in patients with chronic renal failure using semipermeable microcapsules (artificial cells) formed from membrane-coated activated charcoal. Trans. Amer. Soc. Artif. Internal Organs, 17, 246, 1971.

15. Chang, T.M.S., Gonda, A., Dirks, J.H., Coffey, J.F. and Burns, T., ACAC microcapsule artificial kidney for the long term and short term management of eleven patients with chronic renal failure. Trans. Amer. Soc. Artif. Internal Organs, 18, 465-472, 1972.

16. Chang, T.M.S., Chirito, E., Barre, P., Cole, C. and Hewish, M., Clinical performance characteristics of a new combined system for simultaneous hemoperfusion-hemodialysis-ultrafiltration in series. Trans. Amer. Soc. Artif. Internal Organs, 21, 502-508, 1975.

17. Stefoni, S., Coli, L., Feliciangeli, G., Baldrati, L. and Bonomini, V., Regular hemoperfusion in regular dialysis treatment. A long-term study. Int. J. Artif. Organs, 3, 348, 1980.

18. Chang, T.M.S., Chirito, E. Barre, P., Cole, C., Lister, C. and Resurreccion, E., Long-term clinical assessment of combined ACAC hemoperfusion-ultrafiltration in uremia. Artif. Organs, 3, 127-131, 1979.

19. Chang, T.M.S., Barre, P., Kuruvilla, S., Messier, D., Man, M.K. and Resurreccion, E., Phase 1 clinical trial of a new composite artificial kidney combining hemodialysis with hemoperfusion. Trans. Amer. Soc. Artif. Internal Organs, 28, 43-48, 1982.

20. Chang, T.M.S., Coffey, J.F., Lister, C., Taroy, E. and Stark, A. Methaqualone, methyprylone, and glutethimide clearance by the ACAC microcapsule artificial kidney: in vitro and in patients with acute intoxication. Trans. Amer. Soc. Artif. Internal Organs, 19, 87-91, 1973.

21. Chang, T.M.S., Espinosa-Melendez, E., Francoeur, T.E. and Eade, N.R., Albumin-collodion activated coated charcoal hemoperfusion in the treatment of severe theophylline intoxication in a 3-year-old patient. Pediatric, 65, 811-814, 1980.

22. Rosenbaum, J.L., Experience with resin hemoperfusion. In Artificial Kidney, Artificical Liver, and Artificial Cells (Chang, T.M.S., ed.) Plenum Press, New York, 1978, 214-217.

23. Chang, T.M.S., Haemoperfusion over microencapsulated adsorbent in a patient with hepatic coma. Lancet, ii, 1371-1372, 1972.

24. Chirito, E., Reiter, B., Lister, C. and Chang, T.M.S., Artificial liver" the effect of ACAC microencapsulated charcoal hemoperfusion on fulminant hepatic failure. Artif. Organs, 1(1), 76-83, 1977.

25. Chang, T.M.S., Lister, C., Chirito, E., O'Keefe, P. and Resurreccion, E., Effects of hemoperfusion rate and time of initiation of ACAC charcoal hemoperfusion on the survival of fulminant hepatic failure rats. Trans. Amer. Soc. Artif. Internal Organs, 24, 243-245, 1978.

26. Mohsini, K., Lister, C. and Chang, T.M.S., The effects of homologous cross-circulation and in situ liver perfusion on fulminant hepatic failure rats. Artif. Organs, 4, 171-175, 1980.

27. Tabata, Y. and Chang, T.M.S., Comparisons of six artificial liver support regimes in fulminant hepatic coma rats. Trans. Amer. Soc. Artif. Internal Organs, 26, 394-399, 1980.

28. Chang, T.M.S., Hemoperfusion, exchange transfusion, cross circulation, liver perfusion, hormones and immobilized enzymes. In Artificial Liver Support (Brunner & Schmidt, eds.) Springer-Verlag, Berlin, 1981, 126.

29. Gimson, A.E.S., Braude, S., Mellon, P.J. and Canalese, J., Earlier charcoal haemoperfusion in fulminant hepatic failure. Lancet, Sept.25, 681683, 1982.

30. Chang, T.M.S., Earlier Haemoperfusion in fulminant hepatic failure. Lancet, Nov.6, 1982.

31. Shi, Z.Q. and Chang, T.M.S., Effects of hemoperfusion on blood and brain levels of tyrosine and middle molecules. Trans. Amer. Soc. Artif. Internal Organs, 28, 205-209, 1982.

32. Chang, T.M.S., Malouf, C. and Resurreccion, E., Artificial cells containing multienzyme systems for the sequential conversion of urea into ammonia, glutamate, then alanine. Artif. Organs, 3, S284-S287, 1979.

33. Terman, D.S., Tavel, T., Petty, D., Racic, M.R. and Buffaloe, G., Specific removal of antibody by extracorporeal circulation over antigen immobilized in collodion charcoal. Clin. Exp. Immunol., 28, 180, 1977.

34. Chang, T.M.S., Blood compatible coating of synthetic immunoadsorbents. Trans. Amer. Soc. Artif. Internal Organs, 26, 546-549, 1980.

35. Yu, Y.T. and Chang, T.M.S., Ultrathin lipid-polymer membrane microcapsules containing multienzymes, cofactors and substrates for multistep enzyme reactions, FEBS Letters, 125(1), 94-96, 1981.

36. Lim, F. and Sun, A.M., Microencapsulated islets as bioartificial endocrine pancreas. Science, 210, 908, 1980.

37. Bulletin on Tissue Microencapsulation, Damon Corporation, Needham Heights, Mass, 1981.

RECEIVED April 23, 1984

12

Infected Skin Wounds in Rodents
Treatment with a Hydrogel Paste Containing Silver Nitrate

P. Y. WANG

Laboratory of Chemical Biology, Institute of Biomedical Engineering, Faculty of Medicine, University of Toronto, Ontario, Canada M5S 1A8

>A hydrogel paste was prepared by cross-linking clinical grade dextran with epichlorohydrin. When applied to clean, partial thickness rodent skin wounds, this paste formed a protective layer to reduce fluid loss, prevent eschar formation, and minimize wound contraction. For P. aeruginosa infected wound, $AgNO_3$ was mixed to obtain a milky white paste which later became a non-staining, soft brown coating on wound surface. The preparation could adequately absorb wound exudates and reduce evaporative loss. Partial thickness dorsal skin wound, 3x3.5 cm^2, was created on anesthetized Wistar rats by dissection, and then infected with 10^9 bacteria/cm^2. If the $AgNO_3$-dextran paste was applied to the infected wound after 24 hr, healing was delayed. At day 6, high bacteria counts were obtained in separated eschar and sometimes also in internal organs similar to infected controls using plain paste. However, when the medicated paste was applied within hours after infection, the wound healed as uninfected controls in about 10 days, and sequential samplings of the healing wound surface showed few viable organisms. The internal organs were also sterile. Therefore to be effective, the $AgNO_3$-dextran hydrogel paste should be applied to the wound surface soon after injury.

Skin is a multi-layered structure. Its resistance to the penetration of harmful substances and to the loss of vital body fluids by evaporation rests essentially with the outermost

0097-6156/84/0256-0181$06.00/0
© 1984 American Chemical Society

stratum corneum layer which is a heterogeneous tissue comprised of dead, keratinized, partially desicated epidermal cells, extractable lipids, etc. Damage to this layer results in evaporative loss which initiates a series of body physiological changes as well as in bacterial ingress which causes substantial healing delay due to toxins and enzymes released. Therefore, restoring the barrier is an important initial step in the complex scheme of skin injury treatment.

Many dressings have been used to serve as a temporary barrier until natural healing occurs or until the wound site is ready to receive an autograft. At present, commercially available dressings include cotton gauze coated with petrolatum or sulfur-petrolatum mixtures, non-adherent perforated plastic sheets with inner absorbent materials, absorbent fabric pads with a thin aluminum layer, water vapor permeable polyurethane sheets, nylon velour backed with a silicone membrane, etc. In addition, there are many new dressings in the developmental stages (1, 2).

Recently, highly absorbent, cross-linked dextran beads have been introduced in the treatment of skin defects due to perivascular diseases (3). The clinical results have been reported to be very promising, apparently because the dextran beads absorbed exudates quickly which reduced the chances for further bacterial growth and probably also helped to expedite wound healing. The beads are made by epichlorohydrin cross-linking of an aqueous alkaline dextran emulsion in toluene (4). For extensive or irregular skin wounds, it is desirable to have sheets or tacky pastes of the cross-linked dextran material. These materials have been made and characterized as briefly reported in the previous Symposium held in March 1980 at Houston (5). The present study evaluates the performance of a cross-linked dextran paste containing 1% $AgNO_3$ on infected rodent skin wounds.

Experimentals

Materials. Clinical grade dextran was purchased from Dextran Products Limited, Toronto. Epichlorohydrin used for preparing the hydrogel paste was supplied by Aldrich Chemical Co., Inc., Milwaukee, Wis. Concentrated sodium hydroxide solution, the polyhydroxy humectant, petrolatum and silver nitrate are ACS or USP grade products obtained from Fisher Scientific or Canlab Limited, Toronto. The P. aeruginosa bacterium was acquired from the teaching laboratory of our Medical School, and the nutrient agar plates for growth are prepared by our Central Services at the Faculty of Medicine.

Hydrogel Preparation. The smooth and uniform dextran paste was prepared by insolubilizing an alkaline dextran solution with epichlorohydrin (6). After exhaustive washings with distilled water, and homogenization, the solid content of the free flowing thin paste was increased by evaporation to a desired consistency that gave the best handling quality. An amount of 1.25 g $AgNO_3$ was dissolved in distilled water, and added gradually in small, approximately equal portions to 100 g of the paste containing glycerin and small amount of petrolatum, while the paste was being kneaded. The milky paste was transferred in 10-g portions into opaque glass jars and capped until use.

Volume of Exudating Fluid. In order to ensure that the amount of the $AgNO_3$-medicated paste applied will be adequate to absorb the oozing serous fluid from the wound site, a 3x3.5 cm^2 wound was created on several anesthetized Wistar rats (body wt.: about 400 g) by excision which removed thin skin layers to expose the hypodermis. The wound was cleaned and covered with a layer of impermeable plastic film formed after solvent evaporation of an aerosol preparation (Aeroplast; Parke, Davis & Co., Brockville, Ontario). At convenient intervals, the accumulated serous fluid under the plastic film was aspirated through a 25-gauge needle and the volume was read from the gradations on the syringe.

Evaporative Loss Through Hydrogel Coating. Similar wounds were induced on the dorsal skin of anesthetized Wistar rats as described in the preceding Section and the medicated hydrogel paste was spread evenly to a thickness of 3-5 mm. The paste coating extended about 0.5 cm beyond the margin of the wound, and after 4-6 hr when the paste became much less tacky, the evaporative loss of the covered wound was measured over the paste coating with a hygrometer (7). The control was either a similar open wound or a layer of the hydrogel paste spread to comparable thickness on a thin polyethylene sheet and allowed to become less tacky before hygrometric measurements were taken.

Evaluation on Infected Wound. Twenty-two male Wistar rats were divided into 3 groups of 6, 10, and 6 animals. A wound of 3x3.5 cm^2 size was inflicted on the back of each of the 6 rats in the first group as described above. Two animals of the first group of 6 had the dorsal wound covered with the medicated paste about 3 hr after injury, which was the length of time required in later experiments to apply 10^9 bacteria/cm^2 gradually to the whole wound surface. The other 2 rats had the wound exposed for about 24 hr, and then covered with the medicated paste in order to observe the effect of wound desication on subsequent healing or bacterial ingress. The remaining 2 of this group had the wound infected with about 10^9 P. aeruginosa bacteria/cm^2, and after 16 hr, the infected wound was covered with a layer of plain paste. All the paste coating was overlaid with a 2-ply cotton gauze to reduce shifting of the elastic paste due to movement of the animal. The wound on the next group of 10 animals was also infected with about 10^9 bacteria/cm^2 which took about 2.5 hr to apply from a suspension of P. aeruginosa in nutrient broth grown to saturation. After another 0.5 hr, the infected wound was covered with the medicated paste and the animals were returned to their separate cage. For the last group of 6 Wistar rats, the infected wound was left exposed, and then treated with the medicated paste after about 24 hr. At day 6 after injury or at more frequent intervals, the wound surface, the thin eschar layer (if any), and the internal organs were sampled for bacterial content by mechanically disintegrating the tissue in nutrient broth and plating on nutrient agar plates, followed by incubation at 37°C for 24-48 hr and counting.

Results

Exudate Volume from Skin Wound. In the first of the 2 experiments the dorsal skin wound on the anesthetized rat was covered immediately with the Aeroplast impermeable film. Table 1 shows that about 20% of the total volume of the exudated fluid was collected in 1.5 hr, and by 6 hr, as much as about 50% was collected. After 30 hr, the oozing had essentially ceased, and the final volume of 2.2 ml serous fluid was collected in 47 hr for the 3x3.5 cm^2 wound. No further increase in volume was observed even after another 24 hr.

In the second experiment, the wound was exposed for 3 hr before the impermeable film was applied. The fluid was found to ooze much slower and the final total volume was one-half that of the first experiment (Table I).

Evaporative Loss from Covered Wound. The evaporative loss of the dorsal wound covered with the medicated paste was found to be 52 mg H$_2$0/cm^2/hr after 6 hr which was about 50% less than an open wound (7). The value decreased to about 20 mg H$_2$0/cm^2/hr in 24 hr and soon attained an almost steady rate of 12.5 mg H$_2$0/cm^2/hr for the next several days. When the evaporative loss of the paste spread over a plastic sheet was determined 6 hr after spreading by the same procedure, the values was 39 mg H$_2$0/cm^2/hr which decreased to 12.5 mg H$_2$0/cm^2/hr at 18 hr. After 24 hr, it became 7 mg H$_2$0/cm^2/hr, and remained at this level for some time due to the humectant present in the paste.

Wound Covered with Medicated Paste. The uninfected control wounds covered by the medicated paste after 3 hr healed with about 10-15% contraction along the wound margins in about 10

Table I. Serous Fluid Oozed from 3x3.5 cm² Dorsal Wound

Time (hr)	Accumulated Volume (ml)
(Wound covered Immed.)	
1.5	0.4
3	0.7
5	0.9
6	1.0
10	1.3
16	1.5
22	1.7
27	1.8
30	1.9
47	2.2
71	2.2
(Wound covered after 3 hr)	
2.5	0.1
5	0.2
10	0.4
16	0.6
23	0.8
35	1.0
46	1.1
65	1.2

days. The 2 animals with the wound exposed for 24 hr before treatment healed in over 12 days when thin layer of eschar, formed due to desication before the paste was applied, separated from different areas of the healed skin surface. There were also contractions, but wound margin distortion was more apparent. No bacterial growth was found on all the uninfected control wound surface. For the 2 infected controls, 1 died after 11 days, and the other died at day 17. The wounds showed various extent of healing, but high bacterial counts were found on the wound surface and in the internal organs. The summary of these results is shown in Table II.

The animals with wound infected by P. aeruginosa and covered after 3 hr with the medicated paste healed uneventfully in about 11 days (Table III) as the uninfected controls with

Table II. Control Group with AgNO$_3$ Containing Paste on Wound

No. of Rats	Duration before (or for)* Treatment (hr)	Treatment	Healing (day)	Bact. Counts (No./Cm^2)	Observation
2	3	Ag$^+$ Paste	~10	0	15% contraction
2	24	Ag$^+$ Paste	~12	0	Edge distortion + contraction
2	(2.5)* → 10^9 Bact. per cm^2 ↙ 16 → Plain Paste		vary	>10^9 (wound surf.)	Died day 11 & 17

Table III. AgNO$_3$ Containing Paste on Infected Wound

No. of Rats	Duration before (or for)* Treatment (hr)	Treatment	Healing (day)	Bact. Counts (No./Cm^2)	Observation
10	(2.5)* → 10^9 Bact. per cm^2 ↙ 0.5 → Ag$^+$ Paste		~11	~10^3 (wound surf.; day 6)	Some contraction + distortion
6	(2.5)* → 10^9 Bact. per cm^2 ↙ 24 → Ag$^+$ Paste		~22	~10^8 (eschar; day 14)	Some contraction + distortion

minimal wound contraction (Table II). Sampling of wound surface at days 2 and 6 showed <10^3 bacteria/cm^2. The heart, lung, kidney, blood, and liver tissues all gave negative cultures. For the last group of 6 rats with infected wound that had been exposed for 24 hr, wound healing required more than 22 days (Table III). At day 6 and 14, two animals were used to determine the bacterial growth. The healing skin tissue was found to support >10^6 bacteria/cm^2, but the thin layer of eschar, formed due to the 24-hr wound exposure before being covered with the medicated paste, contained >10^8 organisms/g. In 1 rat, the internal organs and blood sample were also found to give very high counts of viable bacteria.

Discussion

At present, the best way to treat injured skin has not yet been established. Some prefer exposure of the wound to form eschar which protects the injured site. Others promote the use of dressings to prevent evaporative loss and to reduce the chances of wound contractions or infection. Most dressings are designed to assist wound healing by incorporating a medicament to reduce infection, using special polymer film layer to prevent adhesion to granulations, having various extent of fluid transmission or absorption to decrease exudate accumulation at wound site, etc.

Table I shows that a 3x3.5 cm^2 dorsal skin wound on a Wistar rat can ooze out 2.2 ml of serous fluid in about 3 days. This fluid volume is reduced to 1.2 ml, if the wound is exposed for 3 hr before treatment. Beyond the 3 hr exposure, there may be further reduction in oozing, but the chance of eschar formation will also increase. Various compositions of the AgNO$_3$-medicated dextran hydrogel paste have been evaluated. The one with a good spreadability and fluid absorption has been used in the present study. Measurements by a simple hygrometric method showed that the medicated paste on the wound reduced evaporative loss by almost 50% as compared to an open wound which had a rate of 93 mg H$_2$O/cm^2/hr ([7]). On subsequent days, the relatively steady value of 12.5 mg H$_2$O/cm^2/hr was about 2x higher than the evaporative loss of the paste spread over a plastic sheet used as a control. The higher evaporative rate of the paste on the wound site might be due to the transmission of excess moisture from the wound surface. The oozing serous fluid had apparently been first absorbed into the paste, because no exudate accumulation was ever observed under the paste coating. The humectant in the paste which retained moisture obviously must have kept the wound surface sufficiently moist to prevent eschar formation.

Uninfected wounds, exposed for 24 hr and then covered with the medicated paste, were observed to require several days longer to heal than similar wounds covered by the paste after 3 hr. It appeared that desication of the injured tissues might have caused further damage to lower tissue layers. On the infected wound, longer exposure before applying the medicated paste also seemed to allow the organisms to penetrate the damage tissues which further caused substantially delayed healing and inferior scar appearances. To achieve the best results, the present study indicates that a medicated dextran hydrogel paste should be applied soon after injury, but preferably after about 3 hr when reduced exudate oozing is within the absorbing capacity of the paste having the optimal handling characteristics as well.

Literature Cited

1. Nathan, P.; Law, E.J.; MacMillan, B.G.; Murphy, D.F.; Ronel; D'Andrea, M.J.; Abrahams, R.A. Trans. Amer. Soc. Artif. Intern. Organs, 1976, 22, 30.
2. Yannas, I.V.; Burke, J.F. J. Biomed. Mater. Res. 1980, 14, 65.
3. Arturson, G. Burns, 1977, 3, 112.
4. Flodin, G.M.; Ingleman, G.-A. U.S. Patent No. 3,042,667 (1962).
5. Wang. P.Y.; Samji, N.; Polymer Sci. Technol. 1980, 14, 29.
6. Wang, P.Y. Brit. Patent S. No. 2,099,704 (1982).
7. Wang, P.Y.; Evans, D.W.; Samji, N.; Llewellyn-Thomas, E. J. Surg. Res. 1980, 28, 182.

RECEIVED April 23, 1984

13

Skin Regeneration with a Bioreplaceable Polymeric Template

I. V. YANNAS, D. P. ORGILL, and E. M. SKRABUT

Massachusetts Institute of Technology, Cambridge, MA 02139

J. F. BURKE

Massachusetts General Hospital, Boston, MA 02114

>Previously we have described a biodegradable polymeric template which can induce wound tissue to synthesize new skin (1,2). This template, a highly porous, cross-linked collagen-glycosaminoglycan (CG) network, is currently used to treat excised skin wounds in patients who have suffered extensive burns (3,4). We now report certain structural and functional properties of the newly synthesized tissue. This preliminary characterization of the regrown organ suggests its close similarity to, as well as certain distinct differences from the intact skin adjacent to it.

The polymeric template was a bilayer membrane consisting of a 0.5-mm-thick top layer of poly(dimethylsiloxane) and a 1.5-mm-thick layer of a highly porous crosslinked collagen-chondroitin 6-sulfate (CG) network. The method of preparation has been described elsewhere in detail (5-7).
    Prior to grafting the polymeric template was seeded with autologous basal cells, implanted into the CG layer using a centrifugation procedure which has been described (2).
    A full-thickness skin wound, measuring 3 x 1.5 cm or 4 x 4 cm, was prepared under aseptic conditions by excising the skin down to, but not including the panniculus carnosus of the guinea pig. The surgical procedure for preparing a skin deficit has been described (8).
    Immediately following excision of the skin, a graft which had been cut to fit within the wound perimeter was placed on the wound bed and was sutured to immediately adjacent skin as described (8). After careful bandaging of the grafted area (8), the animals were placed in cages and were fed Charles River Guinea Pig Formula.
    One week following grafting the wounds were unbandaged and photographed. When the wound had just been covered by a confluent neoepidermis, usually between 10 and 14 days, the sutures were cut off and the silicone layer was removed at virtually zero

peel strength. The moisture flux rate was determined with an
Evaporimeter (Servo Med, Stockholm) after the silicone layer had
been removed. The probe was placed alternately on the wounded
area and on intact skin, previously shaven, about 5 cm away from
the wound perimeter. A simple neurological test (pin prick) was
occasionally administered to the area of the wound and to an intact skin area. Vascularization of the grafted area was confirmed
by observing blanching following application of hand pressure.

At various time intervals, animals were sacrificed and specimens of the wound contents as well as of an intact skin area
about 5 cm from the wound perimeter were either removed for mechanical testing, or were fixed prior to processing for histological
staining. Tensile specimens were stored in physiological saline
at 4°C and were stretched in an Instron Universal Tester Model
TM at 100% min^{-1} at room temperature within 24 h of sacrifice.
Specimens for histological study were stained with hematoxylin
and eosin and viewed in a light microscope.

Results

Not later than 7 days after grafting, islands of new epidermis
had formed between the silicone layer and the CG layer of the
graft, while the host epidermis was invading the area just below
the silicone layer at the site of the wound perimeter. Between
10 and 14 days, the neoepidermis had become fully confluent over
the entire wound area. The neoepidermis formed by proliferation
of the seeded basal cells at the silicone-CG interface became dis-
tinctly keratinized, as viewed histologically, by days 12 to 14.
The collagen-chondroitin 6-sulfate layer was invaded by a variety
of mesodermal cells and synthesis of new collagen fibers became
histologically evident between days 14 and 18. By day 28 the
morphology of the newly synthesized collagen fibers had become
well established in the layer of neodermis. The neodermis showed
histological and clinical evidence of being richly vascularized
by day 7, or earlier. Simple neurological testing gave positive
results before day 21.

A preliminary comparison of properties of newly synthesized
(regenerated) skin and intact (normal) skin shows several close
similarities. However, differences are also apparent, striking
among them being the absence of skin accessory organs, including
hair (the guinea pig has no sweat glands). Figures 1,2,3A and 3B.

Discussion

Preliminary characterization shows that newly synthesized skin
is strikingly similar, though not identical, to intact skin. On-
going studies are directed towards biochemical characterization
of macromolecular components in new skin, detailed morphological
analysis and elucidation of the kinetics of syntheis of new organ.

These preliminary results suggest that the polymeric temp-

PARTIAL REGENERATION OF SKIN

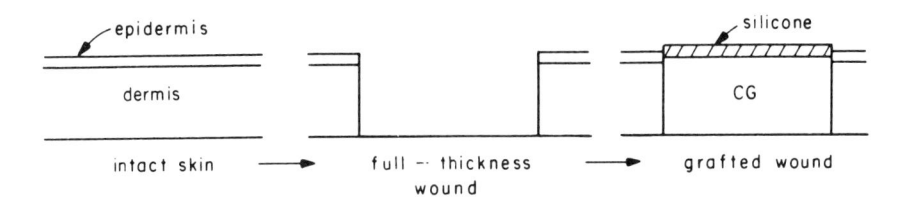

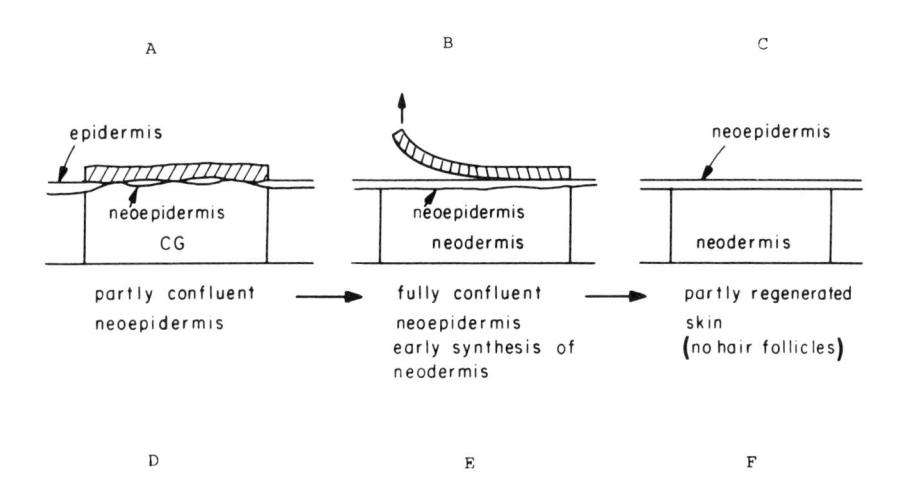

Figure 1. Schematic representation of experimental sequence which led to synthesis of new skin in the guinea pig.

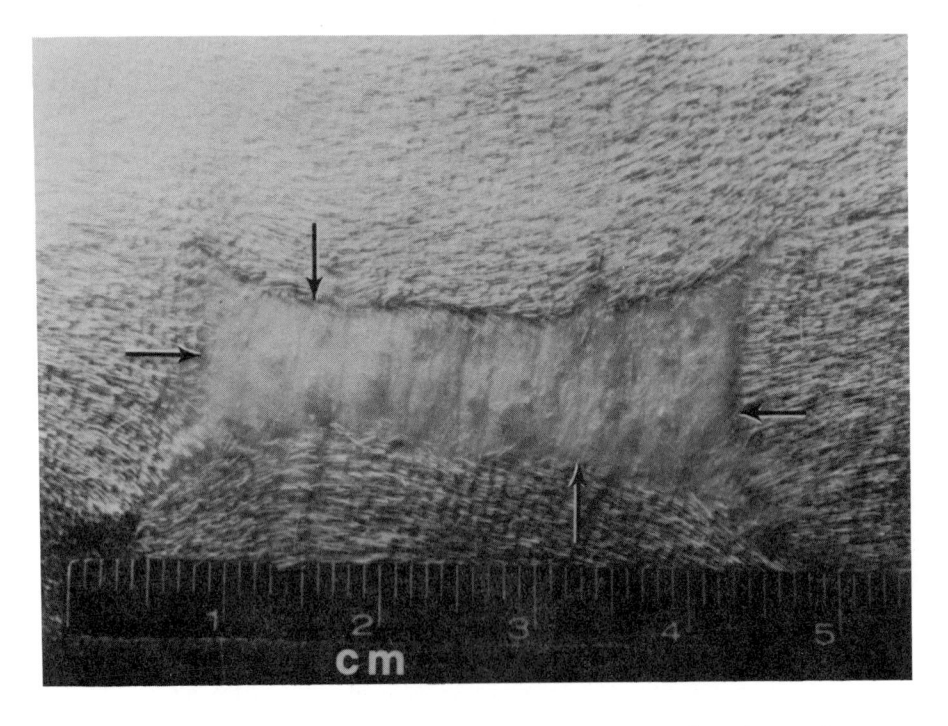

Figure 2. A rectangular segment of regenerated guinea pig skin (perimeter marked by arrows) surrounded by intact, partly shaven skin. Original size of excised, full-thickness wound was 3 x 1.5 cm.

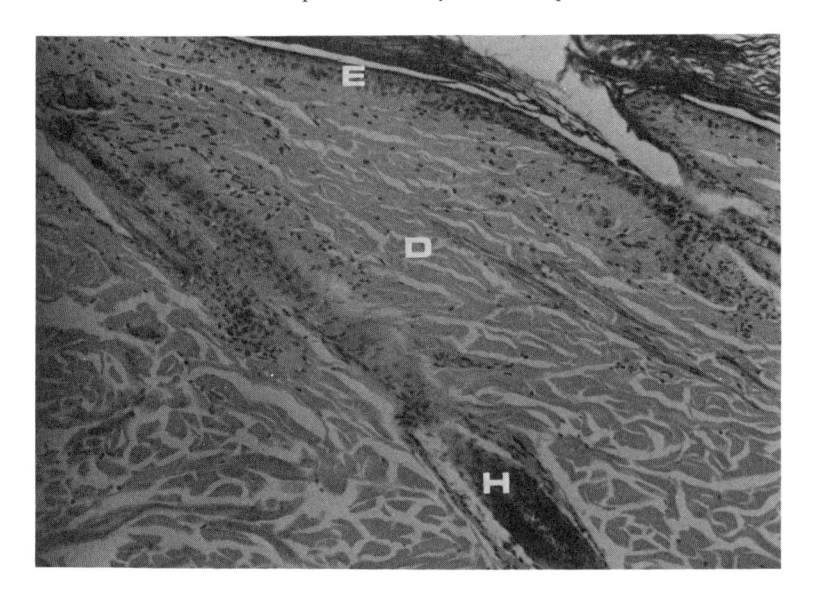

Figure 3A. Histological section of intact dermis. Key: E, epidermis; D, dermis; and H, hair follicle. (Mag. 275X, photograph reduced 15%)

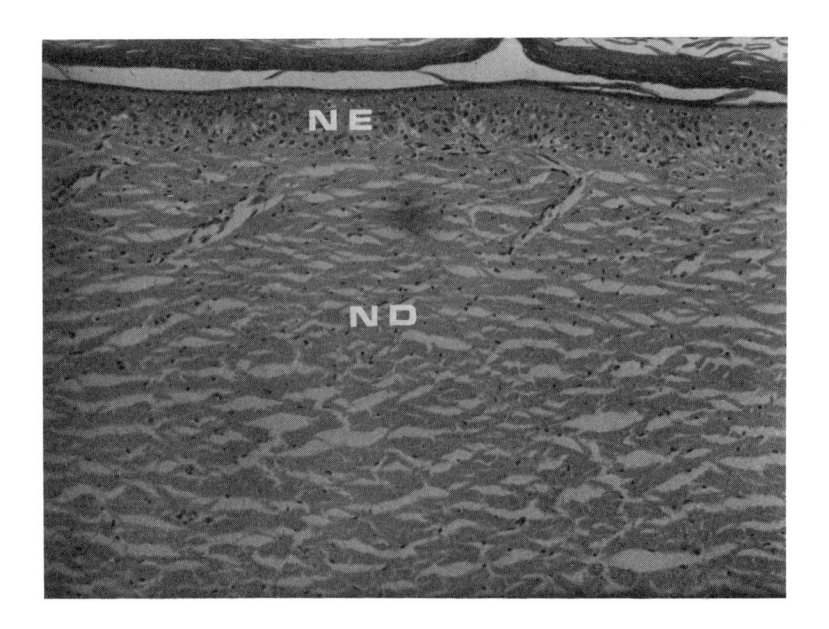

Figure 3B. Histological section of new skin. Key: NE, Neoepidermis; and ND, Neodermis. (Mag. 275X, photograph reduced 15%)

late used in this work stimulates the wounded mammalian tissue in a novel way. The result of such stimulation is not scar, as is the case when this template is not used. Future work will address the question of the extent to which such an unexpected outcome results from repetition of certain late stages of the ontogenetic development of skin.

Table 1. Comparison of New Skin to Intact Skin in the Guinea Pig

Property	Intact Skin	New Skin
Moisture permeability, in vivo, gm/cm^2/h [a]	4.5 ± 0.8	4.7 ± 1.0
Mechanical properties, in vitro tensile strength, Pa	31 x 10^6	14 x 10^6
Second derivative of stress-strain curve	+	+
Histological studies[b]		
Multilayered keratinizing epidermis	+	+
Intact dermal-epidermal junction	+	+
Skin accessory organs (eg., hair)	+	−
Dermal vascularization	+	+
Collagen morphology	wavy	less wavy
Epidermal thickness, μm	20-40	30-40
Dermal thickness, mm	0.8-1.3	0.9-1.4
Neurological test (pin prick)[c]	+	+
Vascularization test (blanching)[d]	+	+
Color[e]	white	white

[a] Measured value remained invariant, within experimental error, between 1 and 10 months following grafting.

[b] Performed 10 months following grafting.

[c] Positive results obtained by day 21.

[d] Positive results obtained by day 14.

[e] Color changes in the graft were as follows: red, up to about 2 months; pink to off-white about 2-5 months; white, after about 5 months.

Acknowledgments

We thank V.M. Ingram, J.C. Murphy, F.O. Schmitt, W. Schoene and D.F. Waugh for useful discussions as well as I. Blank for the use of the Evaporimeter and J.C. Murphy for the use of a Zeiss light microscope. This research was partly supported by National Institutes of Health Grant GM 23946; by the Department of Mechanical Engineering, MIT; and by the Office of the Dean of Engineering, MIT.

Literature Cited

1. Yannas, I.V. and Burke, J.F. J. Biomed. Mater. Res. 1980, 14, 65-81.
2. Yannas, I.V., Burke, J.F., Orgill, D.P. and Skrabut, E.M. Science, 1982, 215, 174.
3. Burke, J.F., Yannas, I.V., Quinby, W.C. Bondoc, C.C. and Jung, W.K. Ann. Surg., 1981, 194, 413.
4. Yannas, I.V., Burke, J.F., Warpehoski, M. Stasikelis, P. Skrabut, E.M., Orgill, D. and Giard, D.J. Trans. Am. Soc. Artif. Org. 1982, 27, 19.
5. Yannas, I.V., Burke, J.F., Gordon, P.L., Huang, C. and Rubenstein, R.H. J. Biomed. Mater. Res. 1980, 14, 107-131.
6. Yannas, I.V., Burke, J.F., Huang, C. and Gordon, P.L. Polymer Prepr. Am. Chem. Soc. 1975, 16(2), 209-214.
7. Dagalakis, N. Flink, J, Stasikelis, P. Burke, J.F. and Yannas, I.V. J. Biomed. Mater. Res. 1980, 14, 511-528.
8. Yannas, I.V., "The Surgical Wound", Dineen, P. Ed.; Lea and Febiger, Philadelphia, 1981, Chap. 15, p. 171.

RECEIVED March 19, 1984

Author Index

Baier, Robert E., 39
Berry, D. B., 99
Brash, J. L., 45
Burke, J. F., 191
Chambers, C., 31
Chan, B. M. C., 45
Chang, Thomas Ming Swi, 171
Franch, R. H., 111
Frisch, E. E., 63
Gebelein, Charles G., 1
Gray, Don N., 151
Harrison, E. C., 111
Hoffman, Allan S., 13
Lee, H. B., 99
Murabayashi, S., 163
Nose, Y., 163
Orgill, D. P., 191
Quach, H., 99
Skrabut, E. M., 191
Stith, W. J., 99
Uniyal, S., 45
Wang, P. Y., 31, 181
Yannas, I. V., 191
Yoganathan, Ajit P., 111
Yu, A., 45

Subject Index

A

Acquired immune system, discussion, 32
Adsorption
 fibrinogen-glass interactions, 55-59
 glass
  ternary fibrinogen system, 58f
  various mixtures of albumin and fibrinogen, 56f
 isotherm and kinetics, fibrinogen-glass interactions, 46-50
Albumin, adsorption, fibrinogen-glass interactions, 55t,57
Aldehyde treated biological substances, improvement of blood compatibility, 168
Analytical sensitivity, antibody detection methods, 34t
Annular vortex, Starr-Edwards ball valves, 121
Antibody detection methods, immune response, 33-36
Antigenic biomedical polymers, immune response, 35t
Applications, medical grade silicone elastomers, 70-90
Arthroplasty, implant resection, reconstruction, 72f-77f
Artificial organs
 blood compatibility, 163-69
 cells, discussion, 171-76
 heart, total, discussion, 6
 immune response, 31-37
 kidney, artificial cells, 173
 liver, artificial cells, 174
 lungs
  discussion, 8
  polymeric membranes, 151-60
 review, 1-11
 role of artificial cells, 172
 silicones, 63-96
Autogenous tissue, overgrowth, heart valve prostheses, 117

B

B-cells, immune response, 32
Bacterial infection, transient leukopenia during hemodialysis, 167

Ball valves, Starr-Edwards, discussion, heart valve prostheses, 117
Ball-and-cage heart valves, with silicone elastomer balls, 92f
Beall disc valve, discussion, heart valve prostheses, 126
Binding, fibrinogen-glass interactions, 47
Bioadhesive phenomena, biomedical polymers, 40-42
Biocompatibility materials in artificial organs, 163
  elastomer, finger joint prosthesis, 102
  medical grade silicone elastomers, 68
Biofunctionality, materials in artificial organs, 163
Biolization concept, effect on leukopenia and complement system, 168
Biological biomaterial interactions, important factors, 22t
Biological cells in artificial cells, 176
Biological responses, synthetic polymeric biomaterials, 23-25
Biological substances, aldehyde treated, improvement of blood compatibility, 168
Biologically active polymers, discussion, 15
Biologically functioning molecules, immobilization in polymeric biomaterials, 19
Biomaterial
  interface, material and surface properties, 22t
  surface composition characterization, 23,24f
  synthetic polymeric, 13-28
Biomedical polymers, interfacial factors, 39-42
Biomeric joint, finger prosthesis, 100f
Bion elastomer, implantable finger joint prosthesis, 99-109
Bioreplaceable polymeric template, skin regeneration, 191-96
Bjork-Shiley tilting disc valve, heart valve prosthesis, 129
Blood
  compatibility, artificial organs, 163-69
  fibrinogen-glass interactions, 57
  response to foreign materials, 25,26f
Blood vessel replacement, discussion, 6
Breast reconstruction, silicone elastomers, 84f-89f
Bubble oxygenators, artificial membrane lungs, 152
Bypass operations, coronary artery, discussion, 5

C

Calcification, Hancock porcine heart valve, 136
Carbon, in biomaterials, 14t
Carbon black loading, effect on finger joint prosthesis, 107
Carbon dioxide permeability, artificial membrane lungs, 158
Carcinogenesis, biomaterial induced, 28
Cardiac valve replacement, discussion, 111-44
Cardiovascular surgery, silicone elastomers, 90
Catalysis, vulcanization, silicone elastomers, 68
Cell
  artificial, discussion, 171-76
  living, primary interactions at foreign biomaterial interface, 24f
  sequestration, hemodialysis with cellophane membrane, 164
Cellophane
  blood oxygenation, 154
  membranes, leukopenia in hemodialysis, 164
Ceramics, biomaterials, 14t
Chain degradation, fibrinogen-glass interactions, 52
Chin reconstruction, silicone elastomers, 78f-80f
Cloth-covered valves, heart valve prostheses, 117
Clots, Kay-Shiley disc valve, 124
Collagen fibrosis, biological response to foreign material, 25
Collagen scar tissue, biological response to foreign material, 23
Competitive adsorption, fibrinogen-glass interactions, 55-58
Complement activation, transient leukopenia during hemodialysis, 165,167
Composite biomaterials, discussion, 14t

INDEX

Composite track valve prostheses, Starr-Edwards, 117
Composition, bion polymer, finger joint prosthesis, 103
Concepts, immune system, 32
Contact lenses, discussion, 8
Coronary artery bypass operations, discussion, 5
Correction of detached retina, silicone elastomers, 91f
Cross-linking
 elastomer for finger joint prosthesis, 105
 silicone elastomers, 68
Cure time, various bion elastomers, 107t

D

Degradation, fibrinogen-glass interactions, 54
Desorption, fibrinogen from glass, 50f
Detached retina, correction by silicone elastomers, 91f
Dextran hydrogel with AgNO3, skin-wound treatment, 181-89
Dialyzer reuse, effect on leukopenia and complement system, 168
Disc oxygenators, artificial membrane lungs, 152
Dispersion, bion elastomer finger joint prosthesis, 105
Disposable hypodermics, lubricated with silicone fluid, 94f, 95f
Drug delivery systems, synthetic polymeric biomaterials, 19
Drug poisoning, hemoperfusion using artificial cells, 173

E

Ear restoration
 discussion, 8
 silicone elastomers, 81f-83f
Elastomer, implantable bion, finger joint prosthesis, 99-109
Electrolyte concentration, fibrinogen-glass interactions, 47
Eluted protein, fibrinogen-glass interactions, structural status, 52-55
Endothelial tissue lining, damage, heart valve prostheses, 112
Enzyme system, artificial cells, 175

Eschar formation, skin wounds, 188
Ethylene-propylenediene-terpolymer, finger joint prosthesis, 99-109
Evaporative loss
 skin-wound treatment, 185
 through hydrogel coating, 183
Extracorporeal devices, artificial membrane lungs, 151
Extraction of polymer additives, synthetic biomaterials, 15
Extravascular system, biological response to foreign material, 23
Exudating fluid, volume, skin-wound treatment, 183, 184

F

Fibrinogen
 adsorption onto various surfaces, 55t
 degradation, fibrinogen-glass interactions, 54
Fibrinogen-glass interactions, discussion, 45-60
Filler dispersion, comparison, bion elastomer, 106f
Finger joint prosthesis
 biocompatibility, 102
 biomeric, 100f
 effect of carbon black loading, 107
 elastomer cross-linking, 105
 Niebauer, 100f
 silicone elastomer, 72f-77f
 Swanson, 100f
 various materials, 99-109
Flaw propagation resistance, silicone elastomers, 69
Flex life
 finger joint prosthesis, 101
 silicone elastomers, 70
 various bion elastomers, 107t
Flexible hinge finger joint prosthesis, silicone elastomer, 72f-77f
Flow visualization studies
 Bjork-Shiley tilting disc valve, 131
 Hancock porcine valve, 137
 Kay-Shiley disc valve, 125
 St. Jude bi-leaflet valve, 140
 Starr-Edwards ball valves, 121
Fluid dynamic studies, in vitro, heart valve prostheses, 114
Fluorocarbon emulsion, artificial red blood cells, 172
Free radical graft polymerization, synthetic biomaterials, 19

G

Gas transfer capabilities, artificial membrane lungs, 158
Gastrointestinal tract, replacement, discussion, 8
Gel electrophoresis, fibrinogen-glass interactions, 53f
Glass, definition, fibrinogen-glass interactions, 45
Granulocyte aggregates, transient leukopenia, 165
Granulocyte function impairment, transient leukopenia during hemodialysis, 167

H

Hancock porcine valve, discussion, heart valve prostheses, 133
Hapten, immune response, 32
Hearing, restoration, discussion, 8
Heart, artificial, discussion, 6,7
Heart valves
  prosthetic, current status, 111-44
  replacement, discussion, 5
  α-Helix content, fibrinogen-glass interactions, 52
Hemagglutination, antibody detection methods, polymeric materials, 33
Hemodialysis, transient leukopenia, 163-69
Hemoglobin, microencapsulated, artificial cells, 172
Hemolysis
  antibody detection methods, 33
  Beall disc valve, 126
  Bjork-Shiley tilting disc valve, 130
  heart valve prostheses, 115
  Hancock porcine valve, 135
  Kay-Shiley disc valve, 124
  St. Jude bi-leaflet valve, 138
  Starr-Edwards ball valves, 119
Hemoperfusion
  artificial kidney, 173
  effect in hepatic coma, 174
  treatment for drug poisoning, 173
  various immunosorbent systems, 175
Hemorrhagic tendency, transient leukopenia during hemodialysis, 167
Hepatic coma, hemoperfusion, 174
Hexsyn, finger joint prosthesis, 99-109
Histological studies, skin-wound treatment with template, 196t
Hydrocephalus shunt, silicone elastomer, 65,66f,67f
Hydrogel, dextran, with AgNO3, skin-wound treatment, 181-89
Hydrogen preparation, skin injury treatment, 182
Hydrophobic interactions, fibrinogen-glass interactions, 47
Hypodermic, disposable, lubricated with silicone fluid, 94f,95f
Hypoxia, transient leukopenia during hemodialysis, 167

I

Immune response, artificial organs, 31-37
Immunosorbent, artificial cells, 175
Implants, various, silicone elastomers, 72-89
In vitro fluid dynamic studies, heart valve prostheses, 114,115
In vitro results
  Beall disc valve, 128
  Bjork-Shiley tilting disc valve, 130
  Hancock porcine valve, 136
  Kay-Shiley disc valve, 125
  St. Jude bi-leaflet valve, 140
  Starr-Edwards ball valves, 121-24
In vivo pressure drop, discussion, heart valve prostheses, 115
In vivo results
  Beall disc valve, 126
  Bjork-Shiley tilting disc valve, 130
  Hancock porcine valve, 135
  Kay-Shiley disc valve, 124
  St. Jude bi-leaflet valve, 138
  Starr-Edwards ball valves, 119-21
Infected wound evaluation, skin-wound treatment, 183
Infection, heart valve prostheses, 112
Inflammatory process, biological response to foreign material, 23
Infusion pumps, polymeric, 7
Insulin level, infusion pumps, 7
Interactions
  biologic-biomaterial, important factors, 22t
  fibrinogen-glass, discussion, 45-60
Interfacial factors, basics of biomedical polymers, 22t,39-42
Internal organs, replacement, discussion, 5-8
Internal reflection spectroscopic technique, biomaterials, 42
Intraaortic, discussion, 7
Intraocular lenses, discussion, 8

INDEX

Iodine-labeled fibrinogen, fibrinogen-glass interactions, 59
Irradiation, resistance, bion elastomer, finger joint prosthesis, 104
Isotherm, adsorption, fibrinogen on glass, 48f

J

Joint replacements
  discussion, 3
  finger prostheses
    biocompatibility, 102
    effect of carbon black loading, 107
    elastomer cross-linking, 105
    implantable bion elastomer, 99-109
    Niebauer, 100f
    polymer properties, 103
    Swanson, 100f
    various materials, 99-109

K

Kay-Shiley disc valve, discussion, heart valve prostheses, 124-26
Kidney
  artificial, and artificial cells, 173
  replacement, discussion, 7
Kinetics, fibrinogen-glass interactions, 46-50

L

Labelling, effects on protein behavior, 46
Leakage, heart valve prostheses, 112,115
Leukocytosis during dialysis, 166
Leukopenia, transient, during hemodialysis, 163-69
Liquid polymer systems, discussion, 15
Liver
  artificial, and artificial cells, 174
  assistance, discussion, 8
Living cells, primary interactions at foreign biomaterial interface, 24f
Lungs, artificial
  discussion, 8
  polymeric membranes, 151-60

Lymphocytes, acquired immune system in mammals, 32

M

Material properties, biomaterial interface, 22t
Mechanical properties, skin-wound treatment with template, 196t
Mechanisms, transient leukopenia, 165
Medical applications, silicone fluid, 90
Medical devices, testing and clearance of synthetic polymeric biomaterials, 25
Medical grade silicone elastomers, discussion, 65
Medicated paste, skin-wound treatment, 185
Membranes
  polymeric, artificial lungs, 151-60
  various, effect on leukopenia during dialysis, 166
Metals in biomaterials, 14t
Microencapsulated hemoglobin, artificial cells, 172
Moisture permeability, skin-wound treatment with template, 196t
Molecular weight, foreign substance, effect on acquired immune system, 32
Mouse strains, antibody detection methods, polymeric materials, 33
Multi-site binding, fibrinogen-glass interactions, 51

N

Natural rubber, finger joint prosthesis, 99-109
Natural tissues, biomaterials, 14t
Necrosis, tissue, biological response to foreign material, 25
Needle, disposable hypodermic, lubricated with silicone fluid, 94f
Niebauer joint, finger prosthesis, 100f

O

Open heart surgery, artificial membrane lungs, 152
Ophthalmology, application of silicone elastomers, 70

Oral biomaterials, analysis of interfacial factors, 41
Organic peroxides, in silicone elastomers, 68
Organs
  artificial
    blood compatibility, 163-69
    immune response, 31-37
    review, 1-11
    role of artificial cells, discussion, 172
    silicones, 63-96
Orthopedic surgery, application for silicone elastomers, 90
Overgrowth of autogenous tissue, heart valve prostheses, 117
Oxygen permeability, artificial membrane lungs, 158
Oxygenator
  artificial membrane lungs, 152
  membrane devices, 154
Oxypropylene rubber, finger joint prosthesis, 99-109

P

Pacemakers, discussion, 5
Permeability, bion elastomer, finger joint prosthesis, 104
Permselective membranes, artificial membrane lungs, 154
Phagocytosis decrease, transient leukopenia during hemodialysis, 167
Physical properties, medical grade silicone elastomers, 69
Physiological response, medical grade silicone elastomers, 69
Plasma, adsorption, fibrinogen-glass interactions, 59
Plasma factors, transient leukopenia during hemodialysis, 165
Plasma-fibrinogen-glass interactions, 57,60
Plasmin degradation products, fibrinogen-glass interactions, 56f
Plasminogen activation, fibrinogen-glass interactions, 54
Plastic surgery, application of silicone elastomers, 70
Platelet, mechanical damage, heart valve prostheses, 113
Platelet function, transient leukopenia during hemodialysis, 167
Poisoning, hemoperfusion using artificial cells, 173

Polarity, polymeric biomaterials, 18f
Poly(dimethyl methacrylate), used in joint replacement, 3
Poly(dimethylsiloxane)
  See Also Silicone
  used in joint replacement, 3
  used in soft tissue replacement, 4
Polydiorganosiloxanes--See Silicone
Polyethylene, used in joint replacement, 3
Poly(1,4-hexadiene), used in joint replacement, 3
Polymer
  biologically active, discussion, 15
  biomaterials, 14t
  biomedical, interfacial factors, 39-42
  commercial, potential extractables, 15t
  used in joint replacement, 3
  various, flex life, finger joint prosthesis, 102
Polymer properties, finger joint prosthesis, 103
Polymeric biomaterials, synthetic, discussion, 13-28
Polymeric infusion pumps, 7
Polymeric membranes, artificial lungs, 151-60
Polymeric template, bioreplaceable, skin regeneration, 191-96
Pressure drop
  Hancock porcine valve, 135
  in vitro and in vivo, heart valve prostheses, 115
  St. Jude bi-leaflet valve, 138
  Starr-Edwards ball valves, 121
Prosthetic devices
  finger joint, implantable bion elastomer, 99-109
  heart valves, current status, 111-44
  review, 1-11
Protein
  eluted, fibrinogen-glass interactions, 52-55
  fibrinogen-glass interactions, 46-50
  interactions at foreign biomaterial interface, 24f
Protein-protein interactions, fibrinogen-glass interactions, 47
Pulmonary fibrosis-calcinosis syndrome, hemodialysis treatments, 165

R

Radicals, generation in synthetic polymeric biomaterials, 20f

INDEX

Radioimmunoassay, antibody detection methods, polymeric materials, 33
Recognition, acquired immune system in mammals, 32
Reconstructive surgery, application of silicone elastomers, 70
Red blood cell substitute, artificial cells, 171
Reflux, heart valve prostheses, 115
Regeneration of skin, bioreplaceable polymeric template, 191-96
Regurgitation
 Bjork-Shiley tilting disc valve, 130
 Hancock porcine valve, 136,137
 heart valve prostheses, 115
Relative polarity, solid polymeric biomaterials, 18f
Repeat units, biodegradable polymer backbones, 18f
Resection arthroplasty, reconstruction, 72f-77f
Response, immune, artificial organs, 31-37
Retina, detached, correction with silicone elastomers, 91f
Reversibility, fibrinogen-glass interactions, 51

S

Scar tissue, collagen, biological response to foreign material, 23
Seepage, artificial membrane lungs, 158
Self-exchange, fibrinogen-glass interactions, 51
Sensory organs, replacement, discussion, 8
Serous fluid from, skin-wound treatment, 184t
Sewing sutures, tearing, problems associated with, heart valve prostheses, 112
Shear stress
 Bjork-Shiley tilting disc valve, 131
 Hancock porcine valve, 136,137
 heart valve prostheses, 113
 Kay-Shiley disc valve, 125
 St. Jude bi-leaflet valve, 140
 Starr-Edwards ball valves, 122
Silicone
 artificial organs, 63-96
 films, artificial lungs, 154
 fluid, medical applications, 90
 layer, skin-wound treatment, 192
 oil, permeation rate, bion elastomer, 105t

Silicone--Continued
 rubber
  artificial red blood cells, 172
  finger joint prosthesis, 99-109
  joint replacement, 3
Silver nitrate, in dextran hydrogel, skin-wound treatment, 181-89
Single protein in buffer, kinetics and isotherms of adsorption, 46-50
Skin regeneration, bioreplaceable polymeric template, 191-96
Skin replacement, discussion, 4
Skin-wound treatment
 biodegradable polymeric template, 191-96
 dextran hydrogel containing $AgNO_3$, 181-89
Soft tissue replacement, discussion, 4
Solid, polymer systems, 15
Solid phase RIA, antigenicity of biomedical polymers, 36
Solid polymeric biomaterials, various, 15,17f
Specificity, acquired immune system in mammals, 32
St. Jude bi-leaflet valve, discussion, heart valve prostheses, 138
Stabilized glutaraldehyde process (SGP), Hancock porcine valve, 133
Stagnation
 Bjork-Shiley tilting disc valve, 131
 Starr-Edwards ball valves, 121
Starr-Edwards ball valves, discussion, heart valve prostheses, 117
Structural status, fibrinogen-glass interactions, 52-55
Styrene-butadiene rubber, finger joint prosthesis, 99-109
Sublethal damage and blood cells, heart valve prostheses, 113
Surface, biomaterial, schematic, 24f
Surface composition, biomaterial, discussion, characterization, 23
Surface phenomena, biomedical polymers, 40-42
Surface properties, biomaterial interface, 22t
Swanson joint, finger prosthesis, 100f
Synthetic polymeric biomaterials, discussion, 13-28
Syringe, disposable hypodermic, lubricated with silicone fluid, 95f

T

T-cells, immune response, 32
Tear propagation strength, silicone elastomers, 69

Tearing of sewing sutures, problems associated with, heart valve prostheses, 112
Template, bioreplaceable polymeric, skin regeneration, 191-96
Thromboembolic complication (TEC)
 Beall disc valve, 128
 Bjork-Shiley tilting disc valve, 130
 discussion, heart valve prostheses, 115
 Hancock porcine valve, 135
 Kay-Shiley disc valve, 124
 St. Jude bi-leaflet valve, 13°
 Starr-Edwards ball valves, 119
Thromboembolism, problems associated with heart valve prostheses, 112
Tissue, natural, biomaterials, 14t
Tissue bioprostheses, discussion, heart valve prostheses, 112
Tissue necrosis, biological response to foreign material, 25
Tissue overgrowth
 Beall disc valve, 128
 Bjork-Shiley tilting disc valve, 130
 Hancock porcine valve, 136
 Kay-Shiley disc valve, 124
 problems associated with heart valve prostheses, 112
 St. Jude bi-leaflet valve, 140
 Starr-Edwards ball valves, 119
Tissue responses
 discussion, synthetic polymeric biomaterials, 23-25
 foreign materials, 26f
 silicone elastomers, 68
Toxic substances, evolution, biological response to foreign material, 25
Turbulence
 Bjork-Shiley tilting disc valve, 131
 Kay-Shiley disc valve, 125
 Starr-Edwards ball valves, 122
Turnover kinetics, fibrinogen-glass interactions, 50f

V

Valve areas
 Beall disc valve, 126
 Bjork-Shiley tilting disc valve, 130
 Hancock porcine valve, 135
 heart valve prostheses, 115
 Kay-Shiley disc valve, 124
 St. Jude bi-leaflet valve, 138
 Starr-Edwards ball valves, 121
Valve description
 eall disc valve, 126
 Bjork-Shiley tilting disc valve, 129
 Hancock porcine valve, 133
 heart, Starr-Edwards ball valves, 117
 Kay-Shiley disc valve, 124
 St. Jude bi-leaflet valve, 138
Velocity measurements
 Bjork-Shiley tilting disc valve, 131
 Hancock porcine valve, 137
 Kay-Shiley disc valve, 125
 St. Jude bi-leaflet valve, 140
 Starr-Edwards ball valves, 122
Vortex shedding, artificial membrane lungs, 158
Vulcanization
 catalysts, silicone elastomers, 68
 silicone elastomers, 65

W

Wall-shear stresses, effect, heart valve prostheses, 113
Water flux, artificial lungs, 158
Water permeation rate, bion elastomer, 105t
Water-soluble polymer systems, 15
Water sorption
 biomaterials, 15
 solid polymeric biomaterials, 18f

*Production and indexing by Susan Robinson
Jacket design by Anne G. Bigler*

*Elements typeset by Hot Type Ltd., Washington, D.C.
Printed and bound by Maple Press Co., York, Pa.*

RECENT ACS BOOKS

"Advances in Pesticide Formulation Technology"
Edited by Herbert B. Scher
ACS SYMPOSIUM SERIES 254; 264 pp.; ISBN 0-8412-0840-9

"Structure/Performance Relationships in Surfactants"
Edited by Milton J. Rosen
ACS SYMPOSIUM SERIES 253; 356 pp.; ISBN 0-8412-0839-5

"Chemistry and Characterization of Coal Macerals"
Edited by Randall E. Winans and John C. Crelling
ACS SYMPOSIUM SERIES 252; 192 pp.; ISBN 0-8412-0838-7

"Conformationally Directed Drug Design:
Peptides and Nucleic Acids as Templates or Targets"
Edited by Julius A. Vida and Maxwell Gordon
ACS SYMPOSIUM SERIES 251; 288 pp.; ISBN 0-8412-0836-0

"Ultrahigh Resolution Chromatography"
Edited by S. Ahuja
ACS SYMPOSIUM SERIES 250; 240 pp.; ISBN 0-8412-0835-2

"Chemistry of Combustion Processes"
Edited by Thompson M. Sloane
ACS SYMPOSIUM SERIES 249; 286 pp.; ISBN 0-8412-0834-4

"Geochemical Behavior of Disposed Radioactive Waste"
Edited by G. Scott Barney, James D. Navratil, and W. W. Schulz
ACS SYMPOSIUM SERIES 248; 470 pp.; ISBN 0-8412-0831-X

"NMR and Macromolecules:
Sequence, Dynamic, and Domain Structure"
Edited by James C. Randall
ACS SYMPOSIUM SERIES 247; 282 pp.; ISBN 0-8412-0829-8

"Geochemical Behavior of Disposed Radioactive Waste"
Edited by G. Scott Barney, James D. Navratil, and W. W. Schulz
ACS SYMPOSIUM SERIES 246; 413 pp.; ISBN 0-8412-0827-1

"Size Exclusion Chromatography: Methodology and
Characterization of Polymers and Related Materials"
Edited by Theodore Provder
ACS SYMPOSIUM SERIES 245; 392 pp.; ISBN 0-8412-0826-3

"The Chemistry of Solid Wood"
Edited by Roger M. Rowell
ADVANCES IN CHEMISTRY SERIES 207; 616 pp.; ISBN 0-8412-0796-8

"Archaeological Chemistry--III"
Edited by Joseph B. Lambert
ADVANCES IN CHEMISTRY SERIES 205; 324 pp.; ISBN 0-8412-0767-4

UNIVERSITY OF RHODE ISLAND LIBRARY

3 1222 00240 9343

DATE DUE			
APR 17 1985	AUG 3 1 1993		
APR 22 1989			
DEC 13 1989			
MAR 03 1998			
MAY 3 1991			
MAY 05 2002			
GAYLORD			PRINTED IN U.S.A.

NO LONGER THE PROPERTY OF THE UNIVERSITY OF R. I. LIBRARY